# Praise for *IBS—*

"*IBS—Free at Last!* is a must-read for anyone with IBS who thinks they have tried it all. Many books about IBS claim they are revolutionary; this one truly is life-changing. As a registered dietitian, I have observed first-hand how reducing FODMAPs in the diet can really work to reduce IBS symptoms quickly. My well-worn copy of *IBS—Free at Last!* is my go-to reference for the FODMAP diet; now Ms. Catsos brings us a second edition that is even better than the original, with expanded menu ideas, travel tips and all new Frequently Asked Questions from her readers. Her practical advice and realistic approach to the FODMAP elimination diet is inspiring and empowering; it offers the IBS-sufferer something that is so often elusive—hope!"—*Niki Strealy, RD, LD, Author of The Diarrhea Dietitian: Expert Advice, Practical Solutions and Strategic Nutrition*

"I was just stunned—within two days on your FODMAP Elimination Diet I felt relief. I can't believe that I've been miserable all these years and not one doctor asked me anything about my diet. I had every test in the book and 'eat more fiber' drilled into my head. I was trying to be a good patient and it was just making me worse. It's been two months and I feel like I've died and gone to heaven."—*C.F.*

"The book is full of great information on a new way to treat IBS with diet. It is easy to read, goes through each step of eliminating, then reintroducing, FODMAP carbohydrates, and explains the science behind it. My IBS symptoms improved dramatically after restricting FODMAPs in my diet…The book really changed my life and health!—*C.A. Dietitian*

"Your book, *IBS—Free at Last!,* is a dream come true for my whole family!"—*C.D.*

# IBS

## Free at Last!

Second Edition

Change Your Carbs, Change Your Life, with
the FODMAP Elimination Diet

Patsy Catsos, M.S., R.D., L.D.

This publication contains the opinions and ideas of its author. It is intended to provide helpful and informative material on how certain individuals can minimize IBS symptoms by manipulating dietary carbohydrates. It is sold with the understanding that the author is not engaged in rendering medical, health, or any other kind of personal or professional services. Readers are advised to share the information in this book with a health care provider before adopting any of the suggestions. Readers are advised to discuss symptoms with a medical adviser and not use this book to self-diagnose IBS.

The author and publisher specifically disclaim all responsibility for any liability, loss, or risk, personal or otherwise, incurred as a consequence, directly or indirectly, from the use and application of any of the contents of this book.

# TABLE OF CONTENTS

# INTRODUCTION

What do apples, milk, whole-wheat pasta, sugar-free gum, and hummus have in common? These "healthy" foods all contain FODMAP carbohydrates and can cause symptoms of irritable bowel syndrome (IBS). If you've never heard the term "FODMAPs" before, you are not alone! The FODMAP concept, developed in Australia but still relatively unknown elsewhere, explains why 45 million Americans with IBS are left to their own devices, desperately looking for help with their symptoms while doctors stand by helplessly or—even worse—give them bad advice.

IBS patients know first-hand that the food they eat affects their symptoms, but doctors have been a little slower to catch on. While many drugs for IBS have been researched and marketed, there has been less research devoted to the effects—both good and bad—of diet and nutrition. Many physicians have not moved beyond traditional one-size-fits-all "fiber" therapy for IBS. It may come as a huge surprise that the high-fiber diet with fiber supplements, beloved by doctors everywhere, usually doesn't work. In fact, if 33 IBS patients are told to eat more bran, only one of them is likely to report improvement of his or her symptoms over the next month. On the other hand, diets focused on the types of sugars and fibers in the diet, such as the one in this book, can help up to 75% of patients get lasting relief of symptoms.

Medical workers are finally coming to grips with consumers' growing interest in nutrition and non-pharmaceutical therapies for IBS. Patients are demanding help with food sensitivities and intolerances, and they deserve to get it. If you are looking for help, you can find it here.

## Who Should Try This Program?

Review this list of common patient statements:
- My symptoms occur in my gastrointestinal tract: excess gas, bloating, abdominal pain, flatulence (wind), diarrhea, or constipation.
- My need to use the toilet can be urgent, and I hate to admit that once in a while I don't make it.
- I've had a positive fructose malabsorption (FM) or lactose malabsorption test.
- Sometimes I think I might be lactose-intolerant, other times I'm fine with lactose.

- Bread makes me feel bloated.
- I love fruit and I know it's good for me, so I eat loads of it, especially when it's in season.
- I eat lots and lots of fiber but my IBS doesn't get any better; in fact, it might be getting worse.
- I felt better when I tried a low-carb diet, but I couldn't stick with it.
- It's gotten worse as I get older.
- I drink lots of sweetened sodas or sports beverages, and eat candy, ketchup, BBQ sauce, or honey.
- I eat a lot of sugar-free candy, gum, or cough drops because my mouth is dry (or I am a diabetic).
- I'm a vegetarian and get most of my protein from soy foods and other legumes (that's "pulses" to those outside the U.S.).
- I'm an athlete with very high calorie needs. I have to eat huge portions!
- The healthier I eat, the sicker I get, so I just stay away from fruit, vegetables, and milk products.
- I do not have fever or bloody stools associated with my symptoms.
- I have seen my doctor, and I do not have celiac disease, parasites, Crohn's disease, ulcerative colitis, microscopic or lymphocytic colitis, diverticulitis, endometriosis, or cancer.
- My Crohn's or ulcerative colitis is supposedly in remission, but I still have symptoms.

Do any of these statements describe your diet or symptoms? If so, this book is for you. It's time to go ahead and get your hopes up! Yes, the low-FODMAP diet has been proven to work for up to 75% of people like you! Those are great odds.

Of course, FODMAPs aren't the answer for everyone. The first item on the above list is very important. If you have reason to believe that your food sensitivities extend beyond the gut, a FODMAP Elimination Diet might not help you, or it might only be part of the solution.

## It's Awkward

My interest in GI health goes back to when I was a 22-year-old dietetic intern at Beth Israel Hospital in Boston. I presented my first case study on a patient, whose name and face I still recall, with ulcerative colitis. As I studied and wrote about the diagnosis and treatment of bowel disorders, little did I know that I, too, was about to be diagnosed with ulcerative colitis.

Almost 30 years later, I have learned much about gastrointestinal disorders, both as a patient and as a health care provider. For me as a patient, there have been good years and bad. I have had enough bad years to deeply empathize with my patients suffering from painful and disabling GI symptoms. Fortunately, my ulcerative colitis has been well-controlled by many years, although I do experience IBS symptoms when I become careless with my diet.

IBS takes a huge emotional toll. I feel hesitant, even now, as I sit down to talk briefly about my own challenges and health problems. How will readers react? Will my symptoms and special dietary needs be taken seriously? Will people think it is all in my head? After all, I *look* healthy enough. It can be hard to get past the stereotypes and judgment that IBS sufferers endure every day. People all too often suffer in silence because of social stigma. These are problems I can definitely relate to, and I am 100% in sympathy with the devastating impact of IBS on your work and social life, despite the fact your doctor may consider your IBS a relatively "benign" condition.

*"I'm 52 years old, yet people are constantly asking me if I'm pregnant! I know they don't want to hear that it's been a week and a half since I had a bowel movement."—C. F.*

*"I feel like I'm missing out on my boys' childhoods. There are so many fun things I can't do with them because there are no toilets available or I just don't feel well. How can I tell them that Mommy has a tummy ache yet again?"—A. G.*

I understand how embarrassing it can be to discuss symptoms, even with a physician, family members, or close friends. I have experienced many of the same awkward moments and difficult social situations that my patients and readers tell me about, and I can really appreciate why reading a book about diet and IBS has appeal as a discreet way to get some help. I hope this book will offer you the comfort of knowing you do not have to face your problems alone.

## It's Confusing

In 2009, when the first edition of this book was released on Amazon.com, there were very few health care providers or IBS sufferers who had ever heard of FODMAPs. In the U.S., *IBS—Free at Last!* broke the story about FODMAPs: what they are, where they are in our food, and how to apply the information. Thanks to the Internet and the rising tide of food composition data being published by researchers, facts about FODMAPs are now more widely available, though the available information is often out of date and contradictory. Sure, it's good to know which foods to avoid. But what CAN you eat? Do you have to avoid all high-FODMAP foods forever? You need a strategy and the tools to carry it out.

This new edition of *IBS—Free at Last!* provides your game plan. I translate facts about FODMAPs into tools that you can use to plan, shop for, and prepare meals. I expect you will find that the foods you CAN eat on this diet are readily available and might already be in your cupboard or refrigerator.

## Change Your Carbs, Change Your Life

Is it worth a few weeks of dietary experimentation to find your way to a life free of that eternal stomach ache and the bowel problems that prompted you to pick up this book? Only you can answer this question; I do know that many of you will find it life changing. I quote here from an email I received from a reader:

*"I have battled IBS all my life. During my 30s the pain and bloating increased. I worked frantically with diet, and exercise to combat my symptoms, but in my 40s, this problem took over my everyday existence. The more I learned about diet and colon health, the more FODMAPs I consumed. In fact, right before reading your book, I was up to eating five apples a day. I also ate tons of onions, garlic, and tomato sauces, never suspecting they could be causing problems. I would often start my day with fruit smoothies.*

*"Today, my symptoms are 95% gone! (Most days 100% gone!) That remaining 5% is truly nothing, and only there when I cheat a little."*

*"This is a miracle! I can't tell you how many prayers I prayed. I can't tell you how many days and evenings I spent on the couch or bed with a heating pad on my tummy. I also can't tell you the enormous amount of time, energy, and money I have spent trying to help myself. I have bought and tried every product that has crossed my path. I have bought so many books! I have tried many, many diets. My dear husband has endured years and years of all of this! I thank you for making my life IBS-FREE!"—B.*

## The Nutshell Version

This remainder of this book describes a step-by-step method for liberating yourself from irritable bowel syndrome symptoms triggered by certain dietary carbohydrates (FODMAPs). You will start by eating a basic diet containing almost none of these suspect carbohydrates. If the diet is going to help you, you should start to feel better right away, typically within two weeks. Next, you will add back one class of carbohydrate foods at a time in a very controlled way. By paying attention to your symptoms, you will learn which foods are triggers for your IBS, so that you can limit or avoid them.

FODMAP is the acronym for **F**ermentable **O**ligo-, **D**i-, and **M**ono-saccharides **A**nd **P**olyols. Don't let this awkward term scare you away! You don't have to be a biochemist to do this diet. I've studied the science so you don't have to. Here is the important part:

FODMAP carbohydrates include certain natural <u>sugars</u> in foods such as milk, fruit, honey, and high-fructose corn syrup. FODMAPs also include certain types of <u>fiber</u> in foods such as wheat, onions, garlic, and beans. (No, FODMAPs have nothing to do with gluten—it's just a coincidence they are both in wheat, rye and barley.)

All FODMAP carbs have a few things in common:

- They may be poorly absorbed in the small intestine. As the hours go by after a meal, these carbs move along into the large intestine.
- They are the favorite foods of the bacteria that live in the large intestine. When bacteria eat FODMAPs, a lot of gas is produced. (Sometimes people have bacteria in their small intestines that can ferment carbohydrates, too.)
- FODMAPs can act like a sponge to draw and hold excess fluid in the large intestine.

With a little imagination, you can picture the combination of gas and fluid causing the large intestine to swell up like a water balloon. People with IBS experience this as a painful bloating sensation. They may pass an excessive amount of gas or have watery diarrhea, constipation, or both. Chaos! I would have liked to name this group of carbs "Chaos Carbohydrates."

The FODMAP concept was originated by researchers at Box Hill Hospital and Monash University in Australia, including dietitians Susan J. Shepherd, Jacqueline S. Barrett, Peter R. Gibson, and Jane Muir. This group continues to publish most of the emerging FODMAP food composition data. If you live in their part of the world you might be interested in the excellent low-FODMAP diet material, shopping guides, and cookbooks published by the Eastern Health Clinical School at Monash University and by ShepherdWorks. The Monash University materials help fund ongoing FODMAP research and can be purchased at the Monash University web site.

Finally, this introduction would not be complete without an overview of the program. This book will guide you through the following eight steps:

1. Educate yourself about FODMAPs, consult your physician and dietitian, and get ready.
2. Record your baseline symptoms.
3. Plan your diet and go shopping.
4. Eliminate FODMAPs from your diet for about two weeks; monitor symptoms and compare them to your baseline.
5. Evaluate your results and plan your Challenge Phase.
6. Reintroduce FODMAPs in a series of controlled challenges; monitor symptoms.
7. Evaluate results and modify your diet accordingly.
8. Enjoy the most liberal and varied diet you can tolerate without triggering your symptoms.

Get ready to begin this short but important dietary experiment! If you can give just two weeks of careful attention to this program, you will learn how your body responds to the change in diet. How much better will you be feeling two weeks from today—50% better? 75% better? 100% better?

The program in this book is not meant to be a substitute for appropriate medical nutrition care. Please share the information in the book with your physician or a registered dietitian and ask for help, particularly if you have other health problems in addition to IBS. You and your dietitian may need to modify the food lists to make them safe and medically appropriate for you.

## A Little about Me

Before we go on, I'd like to tell you just a little more about myself and what I do. I regularly advise consumers to "consider the source" when evaluating information about IBS and FODMAPs, so it is only fair to offer you some information that will help you understand my point of view. First of all, as you already know, I share your history of miserable GI symptoms. I have been in your shoes, trying to practice what I know about the science of nutrition in my own grocery cart, kitchen and body. It is all well and good to know what *not* to eat, but in our everyday lives we need to know what we *can* eat. When we're not feeling well, we don't have the time or the energy to read dozens of research papers and try to figure everything out from scratch.

Professionally, I am a registered dietitian with two degrees in nutrition (Cornell University and Boston University) and experience as a research dietitian and nutrient database manager at Tufts New England Medical Center. My private practice as a medical nutrition therapist has a focus on digestive health, and I see patients three days a week. I spend much of my non-patient time reading research papers related to IBS and FODMAPs and figuring out the most effective ways to interpret and communicate that information to others. I rely on peer-reviewed, published primary sources for my data (much of it produced by researchers in Australia), but I use my own ideas to create tools such as menus, label reading tips, recipes, and shopping lists for my patients. I wrote this book to share these tools with you.

# PART I: THE PROGRAM

**How to Use This Book**

This book was written primarily for lay people without medical training. I have done my best to translate the latest research into terms that anyone can understand. Most readers will benefit from reading the next few pages to get acquainted with the vocabulary and the ideas behind the diet. There are a few big words to learn, but you soon will become familiar with the most important terms.

If time allows, I recommend reading through the whole book so that the changes you are making to your diet will make more sense to you. However, if time is short and you already have a firm diagnosis of IBS, it is possible to jump directly to Step 1, which will help you begin the Elimination Phase and includes menus, shopping tips, and lists of allowed foods. Step 6 leads you through the Challenge Phase of the diet.

At the end of Part 1, an alternate approach is presented, for those who lack the ability or desire to do the step-by-step "learning diet" program. You can still use the tools in the book to reduce the FODMAP load in your diet with this alternate approach.

You can think of Part 2 of the book as the "fine print." Those with an interest in understanding the science behind the FODMAP Elimination Diet will learn much more about carbohydrate digestion and absorption and FODMAPs. Part 2 also addresses the many excellent questions that have been submitted to me by readers and colleagues. You can read this section through as written, or just skim it for questions of interest to you.

Let's begin with the stories of a few patients from my practice who have done especially well on the FODMAP Elimination Diet.

**Could This Be You?**

*Claudia*, aged 52, is 30 pounds overweight and gaining. She has a history of "stomach problems" that goes back to childhood, and they seem to be getting worse as she gets older. She experiences bloating and stomach cramps almost every day and sometimes has explosive diarrhea. She has been seen by a gastroenterology specialist who diagnosed her with gastroesophageal reflux disease (GERD) but found nothing that could explain her diarrhea. He says that her GERD would improve if she lost some weight, but every time she tries to eat a healthier diet—more fruits, veggies, milk and whole grains—she is in so much pain that she ends up going back to her customary poor eating habits. Why does eating right have to hurt so much? It doesn't seem to make sense.

*Mark* was diagnosed with Crohn's disease at age 25. Now 47 years old, he has suffered for years with gas, bloating, and diarrhea. He always has blamed these symptoms on the Crohn's, but recent tests showed that his disease is in complete remission. His distressingly urgent diarrhea makes it difficult to leave the house, for fear of not getting to the bathroom in time. Mark knows he should replace fluids when he has diarrhea, so he drinks plenty of milk, fruit juice, vitamin water, and soft drinks to stay hydrated.

*Dina*, aged 22, goes for days between bowel movements and can rarely have one without using a laxative. She is very health-conscious and makes a point of getting plenty of fiber in her diet. She eats high-fiber breakfast cereal and snack bars every day, as well as apples, pears, and other fresh fruit. Yogurt is another staple food for her, especially when she isn't feeling well. It has been frustrating to find she can tolerate certain foods like ice cream, just fine on one day but not the next. She has done a lot of reading about diets for IBS and has cut so many foods out of her diet that meal planning is difficult, and she finds it hard to keep her weight up. Some friends have hinted they think she is anorexic, but she is just desperate to get through the day pain-free.

*Karin* is 60 years old and has a customer service job. Because of her urgent diarrhea, she doesn't eat or drink anything at all until she gets home at 5 PM, to make sure she doesn't get "caught short" while waiting on customers. She eats and drinks only during the evening, then gets up at 4 AM so she has several hours to use the toilet repeatedly before she goes to work. Her gastroenterologist can't find anything wrong with her. He prescribed an anti-depressant and told her to take a fiber supplement, but she is still having problems.

*George* is a tall, slightly underweight 18-year-old college student with a very physical summer job. His mother does the cooking—lots of fabulous whole foods like beans, hummus, and kale, and plenty of it. He plays soccer for a couple of hours after work most nights—with a pizza chaser. He consumes *thousands* of calories a day to support his energy needs, which means his portions of everything from orange juice to ice cream are enormous. His flatulence far exceeds the norm and his buddies won't let him forget it.

Like the people described above, you may have been suffering for years with painful and embarrassing symptoms. You may have tried all of the conventional treatments for irritable bowel syndrome without relief, or with actual worsening of your symptoms. Eating more fiber, fruits, vegetables, and whole grains does not work for you. It makes you feel uncomfortable or sick. You don't need to be told that "one size does not fit all"—you are living proof!

You may be underweight. Realizing that your symptoms are somehow related to food, but not quite sure how, you may have restricted your diet to the point where you do not get enough to eat.

You may be overweight. Like many people with IBS, you may tend to limit fruit, vegetables, and milk in your diet to avoid symptoms. This leaves you with little more than meat, cheese, and every variety of white bread, pasta, crackers, and potatoes. These high-calorie foods, consumed in filling quantities, are enough to make anyone overweight, which doesn't support your other health care goals.

A few of you, especially those prone to constipation, may have noticed that bread just does not agree with you, "stops you right up," and causes gas and bloating. Have you wondered if you might have celiac disease or gluten intolerance? If that has been ruled out by your physician, you will be interested to know that the gluten protein is not the only part of wheat that can cause GI problems. Wheat also contains a type of carbohydrate that can create chaos within your body. You will learn more about it in the pages ahead.

Can you identify with one or more of these stories? Are you ready to try a short-term experiment to see if you can solve your gut problems once and for all? If so, this book is for you. However, FODMAPs cannot explain IBS symptoms for everyone. Some people have reactions to foods or food chemicals which involve the immune system, especially those people also suffering from migraine headaches, environmental or food allergies, chronic sinusitis, fibromyalgia, or auto-immune conditions. Immune-mediated food and food chemical sensitivities can co-exist with FODMAPs intolerance or can make it worse.

## Swimming in a Sea of Priorities

You may be asking yourself how you will manage a FODMAP Elimination Diet while continuing to eat right for your other health conditions. If you are like many of my clients, you may feel overwhelmed at times by too much information and too many competing nutrition concerns. If you have other health conditions, such as high blood pressure, high cholesterol, or diabetes, a consultation with a registered dietitian can be extremely helpful. Your primary care provider or specialist may have just a short time to spend with you during a typical appointment. Out of necessity, diet is addressed only briefly if at all, as he or she considers your overall medical condition and treatment. Registered dietitians, on the other hand, are medical nutrition therapists—talking about food and nutrition with patients is what we do. Dietitians work with you in depth, helping you set priorities and plan your diet, and providing accurate nutrition information. Nutrition services may be a covered by your medical insurance when provided by a registered dietitian (R.D.). In most states, dietitians must also be licensed in order to provide medical nutrition therapy.

You may not need the assistance of a dietitian if you are in good health except for your IBS symptoms, have seen your physician to rule out other medical reasons for the symptoms, and do not have other nutrition concerns to take into account. In that case, you may be able to work through this learning process on your own using the method in this book.

With the help of this book you can:

- Eliminate or greatly reduce painful IBS symptoms of gas, bloating, diarrhea, or constipation, often in just a few days.
- Learn which types of foods trigger your symptoms and how to enjoy those foods anyway, occasionally and in moderation.
- Eat the most liberal and varied diet that you can tolerate.

Read on to see how it is done.

### IBS Defined—Do You Have It?

IBS stands for irritable bowel syndrome. IBS is clinically diagnosed as "abdominal pain and discomfort with altered bowel habits in the absence of any other mechanical, inflammatory, or biochemical explanation for these symptoms." IBS affects up to 20% of the population. It is more common in women than men, and is often diagnosed between the ages of 30 and 50. It can, and does, affect people in other age groups as well. Symptoms may include:

- Constipation
- Diarrhea
- Gas (rumbling, flatulence, or wind)
- Bloating or abdominal distension
- Abdominal pain

The origins of IBS are not well understood by clinicians and scientists. Over the years, our view of IBS has changed and evolved and will probably continue to do so. At the present time, it seems likely that the symptoms under the IBS umbrella can arise from various combinations of the following factors:

- Abnormal contraction and relaxation of the intestinal muscles that move food through the gastrointestinal system. Such problems may cause food to move through the GI tract too slowly or quickly, and can sometimes cause intestinal muscle spasms to occur.
- Low pain threshold for distention in the intestines of affected individuals, known as "visceral hypersensitivity." This means that a buildup of gas or fluids in the large intestine may hurt the IBS sufferer but not cause a painful sensation to someone who does not have IBS.
- Miscommunication between the gut and the brain, possibly relating to a nervous system dysfunction. Stress may influence these communications in ways that are unclear at this time.
- Low-grade inflammation and immune activation by foods or food components, for example non-celiac gluten sensitivity.
- Imbalance in the community of normal gut bacteria, perhaps in the wake of gastroenteritis, food poisoning or antibiotics.

IBS is sometimes further described based on primary symptoms. It may be described as constipation-predominant, diarrhea-predominant, alternating, or pain-predominant. Treatment usually is directed at the most troubling symptoms.

## Ruling out Other Conditions

You should not diagnose yourself with IBS. If you experience symptoms suggestive of IBS, seek a thorough medical evaluation to rule out other potentially serious conditions, especially if you are experiencing any of the following:

- Passing blood, pus or mucous from the rectum
- Anal or rectal problems such as abscesses, skin tags, fissures, or hemorrhoids
- Fevers or night sweats
- Aching joints or inflammatory arthritis
- Anemia or other abnormal lab results
- Malnutrition
- Unplanned weight loss greater than 10 pounds
- Onset of symptoms after age 50
- Poor growth or failure to thrive (in children)
- Itchy rash or diagnosis of dermatitis herpetiformis
- Family history of Crohn's disease, ulcerative colitis, celiac disease, ovarian or colon cancer

- Foul-smelling or greasy stools
- Incontinence or soiling
- Urge to move bowels waking you from sleep
- Osteoporosis or osteopenia
- Thyroid dysfunction
- Painful urination
- Painful symptoms in tandem with your menstrual cycle

Your health care provider will consider the pattern of your symptoms and compare them to established criteria. He or she will take your medical and family history, physical examination, and test results into account. In younger patients without "alarm symptoms," an office visit may be sufficient to diagnose IBS. In patients with alarm symptoms such as those listed above, a more extensive workup may be needed. If you are a female, especially over the age of 40, be sure that your workup includes a visit to a gynecologist. Bloating and abdominal pain are not always related to the digestive system, even if they occur between periods or after menopause; diseases and disorders of the reproductive and urinary systems should also be ruled out.

Once you have a reasonably firm diagnosis of IBS, you can begin the FODMAP Elimination Diet with confidence.

## IBS in Combination with Other GI Disorders

It is not unusual to have IBS in addition to another GI problem, such as Crohn's disease or ulcerative colitis. In fact, a third of those individuals with ulcerative colitis and over half of those with Crohn's also have IBS. During flare-ups, FODMAPs can be poorly tolerated and aggravate your symptoms. Consult your gastroenterologist before starting the FODMAP Elimination Diet if you have a history of strictures (narrowing of the gastrointestinal tract due to inflammation or scar tissue). Some experts have stated the FODMAPs diet may not be appropriate for patients with strictures.

Crohn's or ulcerative colitis patients sometimes experience gas, bloating, diarrhea, or constipation, even when they are technically in remission and no active inflammation is apparent. If you have Crohn's or colitis, you may get further relief from symptoms during remission by using the FODMAP Elimination Diet. During flare-ups, the diet may help control symptoms while allowing you to eat a diet rich in healing nutrients.

Many of my patients have gastroesophageal reflux disease (GERD) in addition to IBS. While using the FODMAP

Elimination Diet to treat IBS, some of them have experienced remarkable improvement in their GERD symptoms as well.

My point is this: if you are being treated for another GI disorder but are still symptomatic, some further improvement in your symptoms may be possible with the use of the FODMAP Elimination Diet. I advise you to discuss the possibility with your doctor or dietitian.

## Difference between IBS and IBD

IBD stands for Inflammatory Bowel Disease, and should not be confused with IBS. Inflammatory bowel diseases include Crohn's disease and ulcerative colitis. Unlike IBS, IBD causes visible inflammation, ulcers, and other damage to the gastrointestinal tract. To arrive at a diagnosis of irritable bowel syndrome, your physician will first make sure you do not have IBD, which is more serious and requires different medical management.

## A Note about Celiac Disease

Because part of the FODMAP diet involves temporarily eliminating wheat products, the subject of celiac disease is bound to come up and needs some clarification.

Celiac disease, also known as celiac sprue or gluten intolerance, results from intolerance to a *protein* (gluten) present in wheat, barley, and rye. Gluten in any amount is toxic to someone with celiac disease and should never be deliberately consumed by sufferers.

On the other hand, on the FODMAP Elimination Diet, the focus is on the type of *carbohydrate* found in grains. Eating gluten grains does not cause the same type of physical damage to the intestines of the IBS sufferer as it does to the individual with celiac disease. As long as you don't have celiac disease or a wheat allergy, after the initial Elimination Phase of this diet, wheat can be eaten in small amounts, or as much as you find you can tolerate.

If you are still in the midst of a medical workup for your GI symptoms, discuss your plans for this diet with your physician before beginning. Tests for celiac disease are only accurate if you have been eating a diet that includes plenty of gluten. A wheat-free diet could cause tests to come back with "false negative" results. If your doctor plans to test you for celiac disease, make arrangements to have it done before starting the FODMAP Elimination Diet.

## Who Should NOT Use This Diet without Professional Assistance

While the FODMAP Elimination Diet should be safe for most individuals, there are some situations that may require modification of the diet or professional supervision. Please consult your doctor or registered dietitian for assistance with the following:

- Unintentional loss of weight loss or malnutrition.
- Diagnosis of hereditary fructose intolerance (HFI)
- Food allergies or lifestyle choices that lead you to avoid eating entire food groups (e.g. vegans, people who eat "no dairy," etc.)
- Other medical conditions or medications that will make planning your FODMAP Elimination Diet difficult.
- History of strictures (narrowing of the GI tract due to scar tissue formation or inflammation); the FODMAP Elimination Diet may not be recommended for this diagnosis.

## Unintentional Loss of Weight or Malnutrition

I would like to draw attention to a serious concern. If you are significantly underweight or malnourished, you are strongly advised to work with an experienced dietitian as you undertake this diet, to make sure you are getting enough calories. You should be looking at ways to liberalize your diet and increase your protein and calorie intake, not ways to further limit an already restricted diet. You can use the allowed food lists to move in that direction with the help of your dietitian.

## Hereditary Fructose Intolerance (HFI)

HFI is a genetic disorder. Unlike the IBS sufferers with fructose malabsorption (FM) for whom this book is written, individuals with HFI cannot and should not consume any fructose at all. Many individuals with HFI are diagnosed in infancy or childhood, when caregivers note the child is violently ill after ingesting anything containing fructose, such as table sugar, fruit, or honey. Some adults have undiagnosed HFI; they have an absolute aversion to sweet food of any kind, going back to childhood. This "dislike" of sweets may run in the family. If you have HFI or suspect you may have HFI, there are some foods on the elimination diet that you should not consume. Please do not proceed with the diet. Instead, consult your health care provider for an evaluation.

## Food Allergies and Sensitivities

Food allergies and sensitivities also require modifications to the diet. Foods consist of many components, not just the carbohydrates that are the focus of this diet. There may be foods on this diet that you should not eat because of celiac disease, an allergy or sensitivity, or an interaction with one of your medications. Before embarking on the diet, take out a pen and cross out these foods. If you have a diagnosed allergy to any food, you should *not* add it back to your diet or challenge yourself by eating the food without medical supervision.

There may be foods on the diet that you aren't actually allergic to, but which have caused discomfort for you in the past. For example, citrus foods do not contain large amounts of FODMAPs, so they are "allowed" foods on the diet. But there could be other reasons to strike them from your diet. For example, many medications interact with grapefruit and grapefruit juice. Also, citrus fruits and juices are acidic and may aggravate GERD symptoms.

You may choose to avoid items on the food lists that cause you distress for any reason. You always can try adding them back at another time to test your tolerance.

## Medical Conditions

Finally, if you have another medical condition with dietary implications, you should seek help from a registered dietitian to make sure that you do not consume any foods during the Elimination Phase or the Challenge Phase that are harmful or will worsen your condition. Examples of these conditions are gout, kidney stones, gastroparesis, diverticulitis, and celiac disease. Examples of medications that require extra care with the diet are insulin, warfarin (Coumadin), and cholesterol-lowering medications known as statin drugs. This list is not exhaustive. If you are not sure whether one of your medical conditions or medications requires you to limit or avoid certain foods, please consult your health care provider.

## Standard Therapy for IBS

This section briefly touches upon a number of standard therapies for IBS, which have been discussed in great detail in many other publications. It is assumed that IBS sufferers who are reading this book are familiar with, and have tried, standard therapies for IBS. If the treatments mentioned in this section do not sound familiar to you, please take the time to explore other widely available publications and resources about IBS.

Therapy for IBS is usually based on the predominant symptoms. Therapies you may have read about or been prescribed include:

- Fiber supplements
- Laxatives
- Anti-spasmodic medications
- Anti-depressants
- Anti-diarrheal medications
- Stress management
- Exercise
- Extra fluids
- Avoidance of milk, caffeine, fat, red meat, spicy foods
- Choosing bland, "safe" foods such as pasta, white bread, applesauce, and yogurt.

Fiber supplements in particular may be the physician's knee-jerk prescription for all kinds of IBS symptoms. Despite marketing claims to the contrary, recent studies show that only a small percentage of patients improve on fiber supplements.

The FODMAP Elimination Diet is meant for people who have tried standard therapies for IBS but have failed to find relief from their symptoms. Many IBS sufferers stick with conventional therapies for years without noticeable results and become resigned to their symptoms. In fact, my clients sometimes don't even mention their IBS symptoms to me at first. They may have sought medical nutrition treatment because they are overweight, which may be causing difficulties with blood pressure, high cholesterol, or blood sugar. When I hear that they have never been able to lose weight because "healthy foods" cause bloating, gas, constipation, or diarrhea, I know that I have met another candidate for the FODMAP Elimination Diet. Other clients may begin treatment because they are underweight. Progress can begin toward weight gain, weight loss, or other health care goals once disruptive IBS symptoms have been tamed and well-tolerated foods have been identified.

*Answers for the following questions begin on page 91.*

*Q. What do you mean by food chemicals?*

*Q. How can I learn more about food sensitivities that involve my immune system?*

*Q. How can I find a dietitian to help me with the FODMAP Elimination Diet program?*

*Q. My doctor says diet doesn't matter with IBS and I can eat anything I want. Why would he say such a thing?*

*Q. What does the medical literature say about fiber therapy for IBS?*

*Q. Why does my doctor insist on calling my fructose malabsorption (FM) "fructose intolerance"—doesn't he know any better?*

## What are FODMAPs?

OK, I know I promised to keep this in layman's terms, but here comes an awkward paragraph with some new vocabulary. Stay with me, though, because you won't want to miss the rest of this section. It will help you understand how the FODMAP Elimination Diet works.

The diet works by limiting "FODMAPs" in the diet. FODMAP stands for **F**ermentable **O**ligo-, **D**i- and **M**ono-saccharides **A**nd **P**olyols. Specifically, some of the dietary carbohydrates described by the term FODMAP are lactose, fructose, fructans, polyols, and galactans/GOS.   Don't worry about remembering all of these terms. It's more important to understand that all of the FODMAPs have several things in common:

- They are all carbohydrates
- They are sometimes or always poorly absorbed
- They are all rapidly fermentable by gut bacteria
- They can all disrupt the fluid balance in your gut

## How FODMAPs cause symptoms

FODMAP carbohydrates are particular types of sugars and fibers found in certain grains, fruits, vegetables, dried peas and beans, milk products, and prepared foods and beverages. In some people, ingested FODMAP carbohydrates are not absorbed as they should be in the small intestine; instead, they pass through the far end of the small intestine and into the large intestine. Humans have large numbers of bacteria living in the large intestine. This is normal. The problem occurs because FODMAPs act as "fast food" for the bacteria, which give off a lot of gas as they ferment the food. The gas makes your large intestine swell and you experience bloating. If you have IBS, your intestines may be extra sensitive to this, and it hurts.

Another problem with FODMAPs is the way they can pull fluid into your large intestine. This is called *osmosis*. One way to imagine osmosis is to picture what happens when you sprinkle sugar on freshly cut strawberries. The sugar pulls the juice right out of the strawberries and into the bowl. In your large intestine, FODMAPs pull water out of your cells and into your large intestine in the same manner, causing it to swell. Pain and watery, urgent diarrhea can result. In other cases, these changes to the fluid balance and gas production in your gut are associated with constipation.

All FODMAPs are believed to cause IBS symptoms the same way: too much gas and water in your large intestine. It is difficult to figure out what is causing the problem, unless you look at the big picture and take all five different kinds of FODMAPs into account at the same time. All five get thrown into the same "bucket"—your small intestine! If you eat too much of them, they may overflow into the large intestine. The effects are cumulative; the more FODMAPs you eat in one meal or one day, the worse your symptoms are likely to be.

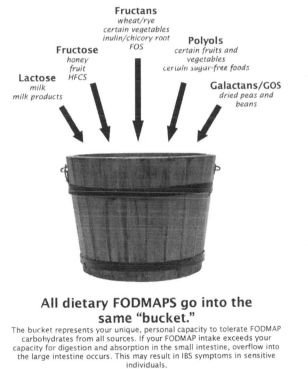

**All dietary FODMAPS go into the same "bucket."**

The bucket represents your unique, personal capacity to tolerate FODMAP carbohydrates from all sources. If your FODMAP intake exceeds your capacity for digestion and absorption in the small intestine, overflow into the large intestine occurs. This may result in IBS symptoms in sensitive individuals.

It can be very difficult to identify trigger foods for IBS without a strategy and a plan. Food intolerances, unlike classic food allergies, do not always follow predictable cause-and-effect patterns. The bucket analogy helps us understand why: all the foods in the day matter, not just foods in your most recent snack or meal.

You may be able to get away with eating something like ice cream one day but not another. On the "bad" day, you may have eaten a lot of other FODMAP carbohydrate foods without recognizing it. You may have had high-fiber breakfast cereal, skim milk, and a couple of coffees for breakfast; an apple and a Fiber One bar for snack; a sandwich, yogurt, and fruit for lunch; and garlic, mushroom, and onion pizza for dinner. That ice cream you had for dessert takes the rap, although it may have been merely the last straw before that belly ache really settled in. Until now, this has made it very difficult to identify which foods are causing your IBS symptoms.

It is the total load of FODMAPs from all sources that causes the problem. The offending load of FODMAPs may be from a large quantity of one food or smaller amounts of several different foods added together over a period of time.

The delay between the time you eat FODMAPs and the time you experience symptoms also must be figured into your detective work. The undigested lactose and fructose in your breakfast smoothie may just be hitting your large intestine around lunchtime, promoting gas and bloating throughout your abdominal cavity. The resulting pressure inside your abdomen might become painful as your stomach expands to contain your lunch. You might wonder what you ate for lunch that caused a stomach ache, but you'd be looking for the problem in the wrong meal.

The FODMAP Elimination Diet solves these problems when the program is followed closely.

## The Elimination Diet is an Experimental Approach

The process that can help you identify your problem foods is called an elimination diet. An elimination diet is not meant to be a diet to stay on for life. It is a diet for learning—essentially an experiment, with you as the subject. The diet is designed to help you figure out whether you are sensitive to FODMAP carbohydrates, and which ones are causing your symptoms. Just as it sounds, an elimination diet eliminates foods that are suspected of causing symptoms in a person with IBS.

The Elimination Phase, described in Steps 3 and 4, is the most restrictive. You begin by eliminating all significant sources of FODMAP carbohydrates in the diet. If FODMAP foods are the triggers for your IBS symptoms, your symptoms will improve quickly, usually within two weeks.

Don't worry, though; you do not have to give up all of the FODMAP-containing foods forever. In the next steps of the process, called the Challenge Phase, you will challenge yourself with each class of FODMAP carbohydrates, one class at a time, by returning foods to your diet in a controlled manner. In this way you will learn which FODMAPs you can tolerate and in what amounts.

If you choose to, you can march through the Challenge Phase in six weeks or so. Or you can stretch it out over as much time as you like.

At the end of the Challenge Phase, you will have the information you need to choose the most liberal diet you can tolerate. You can decide on a given day whether you want to "pay the price" for splurging on a particular type or amount of food. It is up to you, once you are in control.

To learn the most from your FODMAP Elimination Diet, keep the rest of your routine (exercise, fluid intake, and so on) as consistent as possible during the process. That way, if your symptoms improve, you will know that reducing FODMAPs was responsible. In particular, you should not stop taking medications that have been prescribed for you without consulting your physician.

If all of this is starting to sound too much like work, you will really appreciate all of the helpful tools in this book: menus, shopping lists, food lists, and recipes. Even if you don't care to do the whole program, you can still use these tools in a more casual way to help you make IBS-friendly food choices.

**What the Elimination Diet is Not**

The FODMAP Elimination Diet is not meant to be a weight loss diet. The word "diet" is used here in a more general sense, to describe the array of foods that you are consuming. Some people with IBS are in the very difficult position of needing to gain weight, yet having to limit food choices and portion sizes to avoid setting off their IBS symptoms. High calorie intake may be needed for weight gain, or to support high levels of activity such as training for a marathon or working a physically demanding job. If you would benefit from gaining or losing weight, you may be much more successful at achieving your goals after you have used the FODMAP Elimination Diet to identify the foods that you can tolerate well.

*Answers to the following questions begin on page 93.*

*Q. Why do FODMAPs cause IBS symptoms for some people and not for others?*

*Q. What is the difference between a FODMAP Elimination Diet and a FODMAP-restricted diet?*

*Q. My doctor wants me to take a fiber supplement. Which one should I take and when should I take it?*

*Q. Can vegetarians use this diet?*

*Q. I have fructose malabsorption (FM). Does the material in this book apply to me?*

*Q. How does this program compare to the Atkins Diet?*

*Q. How does this program compare to the Specific Carbohydrate Diet (SCD) and the Gut and Psychology Syndrome (GAPS) Diet?*

*Q. How does this program compare to the Paleo diet?*

*Q. How does this program compare to treatment approaches that rely heavily on soluble fiber from food and acacia fiber supplements?*

*Q. Does fructose or lactose intolerance cause depression?*

*Q. Will FODMAPs elimination help my gastroesophageal reflux disease (GERD)?*

# Chapter 1: The Elimination Phase

For those who skipped the introduction, here is a brief recap of the FODMAP Elimination Diet. The goal is to liberate yourself from IBS symptoms possibly caused by intolerance to certain carbohydrates in your diet. You will start by eating a basic diet containing little or none of these suspect carbohydrates. If the diet is going to help you, you should start to feel better right away, typically within two weeks. After that, you will systematically add back one class of carbohydrates at a time. By paying attention to your symptoms, you will learn which types of foods are triggers for your IBS, so that you can limit or avoid them.

This chapter describes the Elimination Phase of this step-by-step program.

## Step 1: Educate yourself about FODMAPs, consult your physician and get ready.

- If you have time, read the earlier sections of this book so you will understand the rationale behind the diet.
- Have you seen your physician to rule out gastrointestinal diseases, gynecological problems, and other medical reasons for your gas, bloating, diarrhea, constipation, or abdominal pain? Make an appointment to discuss your symptoms. Do not diagnose yourself with IBS.
- Review the section entitled Who Should Not Use This Diet without Professional Assistance to make sure this diet is appropriate for you. If you have any medical problems or take prescription medications, this is a good time to make an appointment with a registered dietitian for assistance.
- Review all the foods listed on the upcoming pages. Cross out any foods you cannot eat due to allergy, interaction with medication, or for any other reason.
- As a general rule, do not change the other things you do for IBS. If you take any medications on a daily basis or use any other treatments for IBS, do not change them during the Elimination Phase of the diet. Regularly scheduled maintenance medications should not be discontinued without consulting the prescribing provider.

- If you have been prescribed an IBS medication to be taken "as needed," you can stop using it during the program if you wish.
- Fiber supplements, stool softeners, and preventive laxatives such as Miralax are in a gray area. Although they are sometimes non-prescription, your provider may consider them an important part of your treatment plan, especially if you have a history of constipation lasting more than a few days. It is true that you will learn more from the elimination diet program if you do not take these products, or take the smallest possible dose. However, if there is any doubt in your mind about whether it is OK for you to take a break from them, please consult your health care provider. Transitioning to a non-fermentable fiber supplement or decreasing your dose of laxative may be an option.
- If you already take a probiotic supplement, continue taking it throughout the program. Otherwise, wait until another time to begin taking one, and avoid starting a new probiotic in the middle of the program.
- Unless you are actively treating a nutrient deficiency, I usually recommend taking a break from your multivitamin/mineral supplement during the program. Some nutrient supplements impact IBS symptoms in a negative way and could be part of your problem. For example, large doses of vitamin C or magnesium can cause diarrhea. Some forms of calcium and iron can cause constipation and bloating. Some vitamin supplements, such as Emergen-C, contain fructose or other FODMAPs.
- Consume a wide variety of foods from the allowed food lists to get as many nutrients as possible from foods.

## Step 2: Record your baseline symptoms.

The best way to know whether the elimination diet is working is to keep accurate records. During the week before you begin, monitor and record your symptoms while eating your usual diet. This will be your baseline symptom profile. If you really cannot wait to start, think back over the week before you read this book and write down your impressions of each symptom. In your enthusiasm to begin the diet, please do not skip this step. Without it, you will not learn as much from this whole process. Trust me on this; once you are feeling better, it will not take long to forget how bad you felt just a short time earlier. A paper copy of this Symptom Worksheet can be downloaded from www.ibsfree.net.

**Symptom Worksheet**

Please pull out a pencil and write down the way your IBS impacts your life, using the following suggestions. You can also download a printable version of the worksheet at www.ibsfree.net. Return to your notes at the end of the Elimination Phase and ask yourself how much improvement you have experienced in each category—25%? 50%? 75%? 100%? How much improvement is enough? That is your call.

Your subjective feeling of well-being and satisfaction with your bowel habits are just as important as the "numbers," so be sure to use your own words to describe the impact IBS symptoms have on your life.

**Diarrhea** (frequency of BMs, stool consistency, urgency?)
Before:



After:




**Constipation** (frequency of BMs, stool consistency, painful elimination, satisfying BM, incomplete BM?)
Before:



After:

**Gas/Flatulence/Rumbling** (frequency of passing gas, audible sounds, rumbling?)
Before:


After:



**Bloating** (degree of bloating, tightness of clothing, pain, time of day?)
Before:


After:




**Abdominal pain** (associated with bloating, relieved by passing gas or having a BM, location, duration, intensity?)
Before:


After



Example:

Before: *3-4 watery, explosive BMs most days, sometimes very urgent almost didn't make it to the toilet last Thursday at work, very embarrassing. I feel like my life is revolving around being near the toilet. This has been going on for years but has been getting worse lately.*

After: *By day 3 of the Elimination Phase, I was down to 1 BM per day, stool is more formed. I was able to go for a bike ride yesterday with confidence I wouldn't get caught short. One bout of diarrhea the morning after I cheated and had a big slice of pumpkin pie. Overall, 90% better in this category, feel great.*

## *Step 3: Plan your diet and go shopping.*

Consider writing out your menu for the entire first week. If you wish, you can use or adapt the sample menu in this section for your own use. You can then repeat the menu during week two. Using a prepared menu will help you make sure you have enough allowed foods on hand.

It will be easier for you if your menu is relatively simple, and if you prepare most of your own food during the first two weeks of the Elimination Phase. Focus on reading labels and observing your symptoms, not preparing elaborate meals.

Individual calorie needs vary from person to person. The sample menu provided is not meant to promote weight loss or gain, and if either is desired, please consult a registered dietitian for assistance. If the sample menu seems like too much or too little for you, please adjust accordingly, while imitating the same variety and portion sizes. Those with smaller calorie needs or appetites may wish to eliminate the snacks on the menu. The sample menu illustrates several important guidelines for meal planning on the Elimination Phase:

- On the Elimination Phase, you should eat only foods on the allowed lists and avoid those that are not specifically named on the lists.
- Don't make the common mistake of jumping to the conclusion that one of the categories of FODMAPs is not a problem for you because you eat it routinely. You may be tempted to think that white bread or yogurt, for example, aren't part of your problem because you can often eat them without experiencing symptoms. This may be the result of coincidentally eating less of the other FODMAPs on those good days. Don't make assumptions. Avoid making exceptions. You will learn the most and have the best results if you eat ONLY foods allowed on the Elimination Phase. It's only for two weeks—you can do it! There will be plenty of time for experimenting later.
- On the other hand, don't assume that you are lactose-intolerant unless you have had a positive result on a hydrogen breath test. Even then, you might consider taking the time to check out tolerance for yourself. I have had many clients who have unnecessarily eliminated "dairy" from their diets because they have read somewhere that people with IBS should avoid it. *This is a very common mistake.*

Don't deprive yourself of the nutrients in milk products unless you prove to yourself that you have to.

- Portion sizes are important for some food. Foods listed in boldface type must be consumed in limited portions because they do contain small amounts of FODMAPs.
- Consume only one boldface food per meal or snack. This limits the total FODMAPs load to a very low level, which will be unlikely to provoke any symptoms.
- For other foods, portion sizes are merely suggestions. You can vary them according to your needs and appetite.

Except for the rule to limit yourself to one boldface food per meal or snack, this plan does not attempt to instruct you on how many servings to eat from each food group. There are many other variables affecting your needs which fall outside the scope of this book. Just remember that variety and moderation are the keys to a healthy diet. Choose fewer empty calories and more nutrient-rich foods. With the FODMAP Elimination Diet, you may finally be able to eat the lower FODMAP fruits, vegetables, whole grains, and dairy products your body craves and needs.

## Sample Menus

There are several variations of the breakfast and morning snack pattern which take into account how people take their coffee. If you take cream in coffee (a boldface item) with breakfast, you should hold off on fruit (also a boldface item) until snack time.

To make the menus more practical, there is some deliberate repetition in the sample menu. I assume you will want to use a perishable item—blueberries, for instance—before it goes bad, so you will see it repeated on the menu several times. If you prefer, you can easily make substitutions to the sample menu by consulting the food lists in Step 4. You can also design your own menu from scratch to suit your food preferences. The recipes referred to are provided at the end of this book.

## Day 1

*Breakfast*
1 C. corn flakes
1 C. lactose-free skim milk
**½ ripe banana**

*Snack*
**Small handful almonds**

*Lunch*
2 slices wheat- and rye-free bread
2 oz. turkey
Lettuce and fresh tomato
2 T. real mayonnaise
**½ C. fresh blueberries**
½ C. baby carrots

*Snack*
½ C. lactose-free cottage cheese
8 cherry tomatoes

*Dinner*
4 oz. baked salmon
Medium baked potato
**1 ½ T. sour cream**
2 C. raw baby spinach
½ C. slivered red bell pepper
1 t. olive oil
1 T. balsamic vinegar

*Beverages*
Water or tea, as desired; **1 C. of coffee** per day

### Day 2

*Breakfast*
1 C. cooked oatmeal/porridge
1 C. lactose-free skim milk
**½ ripe banana**

*Morning Snack*
1 oz. rice crackers
1 hard-boiled egg
2 T. half-and-half for coffee

*Lunch*
2 skillet-warmed corn tortillas
3 oz. tuna
2 T. light mayonnaise
Lettuce and tomato
**1 small orange**
½ C. baby carrots

*Afternoon Snack*
1 oz. low-fat cheddar cheese
8 cherry tomatoes

*Dinner*
3 oz. grilled turkey burger
1 oz. cheddar cheese
1 C. brown rice
2 C. mixed salad greens
1 t. olive oil
1 T. balsamic vinegar
**2 peanut butter cookies (recipe)**

*Evening Snack*
**½ C. grapes**

*Beverages*
Water or tea, as desired; **1 C. of coffee** per day

## Day 3

*Breakfast*
1 C. cooked oatmeal/porridge
1 C. lactose-free skim milk
**1 ½ t. sugar for coffee**

*Morning Snack*
**½ C. blueberries**
½ C. lactose-free cottage cheese

*Lunch*
3 oz. grilled chicken
1 C. grilled zucchini
**2 T. slivered almonds**
Medium baked potato
1 t. butter

*Afternoon Snack*
**Granola bar (recipe)**

*Dinner*
1 C. rice pasta
4 oz. roast pork tenderloin
2 t. olive oil
2 C. celery and carrots, stir fried
Soy sauce
**1 small orange**

*Evening Snack*
**2 T. almonds**

*Beverages*
Water or tea, as desired; 1 C. of coffee per day

### Day 4

*Breakfast*
1 C. sliced, cooked potatoes
2 t. butter
1 egg
**1/3 C. orange juice**

*Morning Snack*
½ C. plain instant oatmeal/porridge
**2 T. slivered almonds**
1 C. lactose-free skim milk

*Lunch*
2 slices wheat- and rye-free bread
2 oz. turkey
Lettuce and tomato
2 T. real mayonnaise
**½ C. blueberries**
½ C. baby carrots

*Afternoon Snack*
½ C. lactose-free cottage cheese
1 C. peeled cucumber slices

*Dinner*
2 skillet-warmed corn tortillas
4 oz. grilled steak
½ C. sautéed red pepper strips
2 t. olive oil
½ C. chopped fresh tomato
**1 ½ T. sour cream**

*Evening Snack*
**Granola bar (recipe)**

*Beverages*
Water or tea, as desired; **1 C. of coffee** per day

## Day 5

*Breakfast*
1 C. corn flakes
1 C. lactose-free skim milk
**½ ripe banana**

*Morning Snack*
3 plain rice cakes
1 oz. cheddar cheese

*Lunch*
1 oz. baked potato chips
2 C. mixed salad greens
½ C. mixed cucumber and **green peas**
3 oz. turkey
1 T. olive oil
2 T. balsamic wine vinegar

*Afternoon Snack*
½ C. lactose-free cottage cheese
**½ C. blueberries**

*Dinner*
1 baked pork chop
1 C. brown rice
2 t. butter
**½ C. green peas**
½ C. red pepper strips

*Evening Snack*
1 oz. rice crackers
**Small handful peanuts**

*Beverages*
Water or tea, as desired; **1 C. of coffee** per day

### Day 6

*Breakfast*
1 C. corn flakes
1 C. lactose-free skim milk
**2 T. slivered almonds**

*Morning Snack*
**½ C. strawberries**
1 oz. rice crackers
1 hard-boiled egg

*Lunch*
1 serving Pork Fried Rice (recipe)
**½ C. canned pineapple chunks**

*Afternoon Snack*
1 oz. cheddar cheese
½ C. baby carrots

*Dinner*
4 oz. grilled chicken
1 C. Quinoa Salad (recipe)
**1 small orange**

*Evening Snack*
**Small handful peanuts**

*Beverages*
Water or tea, as desired; **1 C. of coffee** per day

## Day 7

*Breakfast*
1 C. cooked, sliced potatoes
2 t. butter
1 egg
½ C. baby spinach
**1/3 C. orange juice**

*Morning Snack*
2 slices toasted wheat- and rye-free bread
2 t. butter
1 C. lactose-free milk

*Lunch*
1 serving Pork Fried Rice (leftover from yesterday)
**½ C. strawberries**

*Afternoon Snack*
2 slices lean deli roast beef
½ medium red bell pepper, strips

*Dinner*
3 oz. grilled chicken
1 C. brown rice
2 C. mixed salad greens
**2 T. slivered almonds**
1 t. olive oil
1 T. balsamic wine vinegar

*Evening Snack*
**½ C. strawberry sorbet, sugar sweetened**

*Beverages*
Water or tea, as desired; **1 C. of coffee** per day

## Shopping List for Sample Menu

A shopping list for the sample menu is provided below, and can also be downloaded from www.ibsfree.net. Shopping from a list based on your Week 1 menu will ensure that you have all of your allowed foods on hand and help your first week go smoothly.

- Please read labels for all prepared items. For example, "corn flakes" should not have any high-fructose corn syrup or fruit juice concentrate used as sweetener.
- Please see www.ibsfree.net for ideas on brand names if you are having trouble finding what you need.
- Visit the health food aisle of a well-stocked grocery store to find nuts and seeds available in bulk bins. That is the easiest, least expensive way to buy small quantities of nuts and seeds. (If you are on a gluten-free diet do not buy from bulk bins, which are not protected from cross-contamination).
- Items that are for recipes only are in italics. If you don't plan to do any cooking (you know who you are), you can skip them, but you may have to buy more of the other things to last the whole week.
- 

### Grocery Items

1 box corn flakes
1 lb. box quick rolled oats
8 oz. box plain instant oatmeal/porridge
4 oz. chopped walnuts
4 oz. slivered almonds
2 oz. whole almonds
*2 oz. almond flour*
*4 oz. pecans*
4 oz. cashews
4 oz. peanuts
*4 oz. pumpkin seeds/pepitas*
1 small jar real mayonnaise
Small bottle olive oil
*Small bottle Karo light corn syrup (or Lyle's Golden Syrup)*
*12 oz. jar creamy peanut butter*
Small bottle balsamic vinegar
*Small bottle rice vinegar*
*Small bottle low-sodium soy sauce*
*Small bottle sesame oil*
*Small bottle vanilla extract*
*Small bottle 100% pure maple syrup*
1 bag plain rice cakes
Small package rice pasta
Two 3.5 oz. packages rice crackers
Small package 6" corn tortillas
3 oz. can water-packed tuna fish
20 oz. can pineapple chunks
1 lb. dry brown rice
*¾ lb. uncooked quinoa*
1 lb. granulated sugar
1 oz. baked potato chips
1 loaf bread (free of wheat, rye, and fruit juice concentrate)

## Produce

1 bunch leaf lettuce
1 lb. mixed salad greens
2 fresh tomatoes
*Small piece fresh ginger*
1 lb. baby carrots
1 bunch celery
1 pint cherry or grape
   tomatoes
2 small cucumbers
4 medium potatoes
1 lb. carrots
1 small zucchini
*1 cup bean sprouts*
3 red bell peppers
*1 bunch green onions/scallions*
½ lb. fresh baby spinach
2 medium bananas
3 small oranges
*3 fresh lemons*
1 pint fresh blueberries
1 pint fresh strawberries
*Small bunch fresh mint or parsley*
*Small bunch chives*

## Egg/Dairy Case

½ gallon lactose-free skim
   milk
½ lb. butter
Small carton light sour cream
1 lb. carton lactose-free
   cottage cheese
1 dozen eggs
6 oz. package cheddar cheese
8 fluid oz. bottle or carton
   orange juice

## Meat/Fish/Poultry

½ lb. deli sliced turkey
2 oz. deli sliced lean roast
   beef
5 oz. fresh salmon
1 lb. boneless, skinless
   chicken
1 lb. pork loin or tenderloin
1 pork chop
5 oz. beef steak
5 oz. lean ground turkey

## Frozen

1 pint strawberry sorbet with
   allowed ingredients
Small bag frozen green peas

*Answers to the following questions begin on page 98.*

*Q. I don't like/can't get some of the foods on your sample menus. What else can I have?*

*Q. Do you have some meal ideas for vegetarians?*

*Q. I eat out a lot. What can I order at restaurants that will work on this diet?*

*Q. My health care provider wants me to gain weight—which foods on the FODMAPs Elimination Phase would be useful for this purpose?*

*Q. I need to lose some weight. Can I use the FODMAP Elimination Diet for that?*

## Step 4: Eliminate FODMAPs from your diet for about two weeks; monitor symptoms

- Start the Elimination Phase of the diet at the beginning of a two week stretch when you will be able to buy and prepare almost all of your own food.
- The foods can be simply prepared, but if you are used to eating out frequently, you will need to allow some extra time for these tasks.
- Use the sample menus on the previous pages or vary your diet with choices from the allowed food lists.
- For the two-week duration of the Elimination Phase, eat ONLY foods specifically named on the lists of allowed foods that follow. Later, you will be able to experiment with any food you desire, but for the first two weeks, eat only allowed foods, simply prepared. In other words, be aware of sauces and other additions to your food. Make sure they, too, are allowed.
- For prepared or processed foods on the lists, please check to make sure all ingredients are allowed. For example, turkey is an allowed food. You should either roast the turkey yourself (from a bird packaged with no problem ingredients) or ask to check the label on the processed turkey at the deli.
- Limit yourself to the serving sizes suggested for all fruits, sweets and other foods in **bold** type. **Choose only one of these foods per meal or snack**. For all other foods, portion sizes are suggestions only.

*Answers to the following questions begin on page 104.*

*Q. Why is there so much conflicting information about FODMAPs on the Internet?*

*Q. I'm going on vacation next week; should I start the diet now or wait till my holiday is over?*

*Q. How soon can I eat another **bold** food?*

*Q. Do I really have to stay on the Elimination Phase for two weeks if I feel better right away?*

*Q. Don't I need to know the exact number of grams of FODMAPs in all these foods?*

*Q. What about kale, or kumquats, or any one of the many foods that don't appear on the lists in this book?*

*Q. I see one of my problem foods on the allowed lists. I could never eat that! What does this mean?*

*Q. Those portions are too small/too big for me. Can I eat more/less?*

*Q. Do I have to worry about FODMAPs in my skin care or personal hygiene products?*

*Q. What can I use to replace fluids lost in diarrhea or excessive perspiration?*

*Q. From years of trouble with my bowels, I am practically obsessed with getting enough fiber! How can I get enough fiber on this diet?*

*Q. Which foods are the best sources of vitamins and minerals?*

### Allowed Grains and Starches

All of the foods on this list are allowed because they are either known to be, or likely to be, low in fructans. Note that wheat, barley, and rye are not allowed. Corn products are allowed, but not sweet corn. Serving sizes are suggestions.

Amaranth, cooked, ½ C.
Breakfast cereals made of oats, rice, corn, buckwheat, quinoa, amaranth or millet, ½ C.
Buckwheat cereal, cooked, ½ C.
Buckwheat flour, ¼ C.
Soba noodles (100% buckwheat), cooked, ½ C.
Oatmeal/porridge, cooked, ½ C.
Oat bran, cooked, ½ C.
Oat flour, ½ C.
Grits, cooked, ½ C.
Corn, rice or quinoa pasta, cooked, ½ C.
Corn tortillas, 6 inch
Corn or tortilla chips, 1 oz.
Crackers, rice or corn, 14 small
Cornmeal, ¼ C.
Millet, cooked, ¼ C.
Popcorn, popped, 2 C.
Potato, cooked, ½ C. or 1 small
Potato chips, 1 oz.
Quinoa, cooked, ½ C.
Rice or popcorn cakes, unflavored, 3 large
Rice, brown or white, plain, cooked, ⅓ C. (no mixes or packets)
Rice bran, uncooked, 2 T.
Wild rice, plain, cooked, ⅓ C.

*Please read labels carefully, and avoid the following:*

- Wheat as a major ingredient, including wheat flour, white flour, enriched flour, all-purpose flour, and whole wheat flour (check cereals, breads, crackers, pastas, cookies, crisps, biscuits, cake, pastries, muffins, bagels, pizza, sauces, gravies)
- Kamut and spelt, which are particular varieties of wheat (check cereals, breads, crackers, pastas, cookies, crisps, biscuits, cake, pastries, muffins, bagels, pizza, sauces, gravies)
- Wheat berries or sprouted wheat (check breads)
- Chicory root or extract (check cereals, snack, granola, fiber, nutrition or energy bars)

- Inulin (check baked goods, instant oatmeal, cereals, snack, granola, fiber, nutrition or energy bars)
- Fructo-oligosaccharides/FOS (check low-fat cookies, snack, granola, fiber, nutrition or energy bars, cereals)
- Fructose, crystalline fructose, high-fructose corn syrup (check baked goods, snack, granola, fiber, nutrition or energy bars, cereals)
- Sorbitol, mannitol, isomalt, xylitol, maltitol, lactitol, polydextrose, or hydrogenated starch hydrolysates (check low-carb snacks or meal replacement bars)
- Molasses (check baked goods, peanut butter)
- Fruit juice concentrate (check breads, baked goods, snack, granola, fiber, nutrition or energy bars, cereals)

*These ingredients and descriptions are allowed:*

- Corn starch
- Modified food starch
- Resistant starch
- Wheat starch
- Maltodextrin
- Carageenan
- Guar gum
- Xanthan gum
- Gluten-free foods. Gluten-free claims on food labels may help you quickly identify wheat-free foods (although, as you know, gluten is not the part of wheat that you are avoiding). You should still read the label to check for the presence of other problem ingredients.
- Foods "produced in a facility that also makes products containing wheat." A trace of wheat in a product is not enough to cause problems with this diet.

*Answers to the following questions begin on page 111.*

*Q. I'm surprised to see that modified and resistant starches, gums, pectin, and carageenan are allowed? Why is that?*

*Q. Why don't you allow spelt on this diet when other sources say it is OK?*

## Allowed Fruits

Fruits are the most limited food group on this elimination diet. You may be eating less fruit than usual. You can make up for this by eating more vegetables, since fruits and vegetables provide many of the same nutrients.

Fruits with more fructose than glucose are not allowed on the Elimination Phase of your diet, nor are fruits that contain polyols. All of the fruits on the following list are allowed because the fructose and glucose in the fruit are balanced, the total fructose per serving is not too high, and they are low in polyols. Fruits may be fresh, frozen or canned in their own juices.

A note about bananas: as they ripen, the starches (polysaccharides) in the banana are converted to sugars. The sugars are balanced, so limited portions of ripe bananas are allowed on the Elimination Phase. Ripe bananas are also likely to be better tolerated.

The serving size is critical for this food group. Allowed serving sizes are in boldface type. If the total fructose load of the meal is too high, even if balanced with glucose, symptoms may occur.

If breath testing has shown you have severe fructose malabsorption, use even smaller portions or omit fruit altogether for the short duration of the Elimination Phase.

**Banana, ripe, ½**
**Blueberries, ½ C.**
**Blueberry juice, ⅓ C.**
**Cantaloupe, ½ C.**
**Clementine, 1 medium**
**Cranberries, raw, ½ C.**
**Dragon fruit, ½ C.**
**Durian, ½ C.**
**Grapefruit juice, ⅓ C.**
**Grapefruit, ½ large**
**Grapes, all kinds, ½ C.**
**Honeydew melon, ½ C.**
**Kiwi, 1 medium**
**Lemon juice, ⅓ C.**
**Lime juice, ⅓ C.**
**Orange juice, ⅓ C.**
**Orange, 1 small**
**Papaya/paw paw, ½ C.**
**Pineapple, ½ C.**

**Prickly pear fruit, 1**
**Rambutan, ½ C.**
**Raspberries, ½ C.**
**Rhubarb, ½ C.**
**Strawberries, ½ C.**
**Tangelo, 1 medium**

*Please read labels carefully and avoid the following:*

- Crystalline fructose (fruit drinks or cocktails, fizzy drink mixes such as Emergen-C®, fruit jam or jelly, fruit-flavored candy, sauces such as ketchup, plum sauce, or chutney, protein powders)
- High-fructose corn syrup (fruit drinks or cocktails, fizzy drink mixes such as Emergen-C®, fruit jam or jelly, fruit-flavored candy, sauces such as ketchup, plum sauce, or chutney)
- Fruit juice concentrate (check energy or snack bars, fruit drinks or cocktails, fruit spreads, leathers, or gummies, frozen fruit bars, cookies, sweets of any kind with "healthy" or "naturally sweetened" label claims)
- Fruit-juice based alcoholic drinks such as tequila sunrise, sea breeze, piña colada, mai tai, or daiquiri
- Dehydrated fruits in "whole food" type supplements or protein powders

*These ingredients and descriptions are allowed:*

- Pectin
- Sugar

**Allowed Vegetables**

Vegetables containing large amounts of galactans (also known as galacto-oligosaccharides or GOS) or short-chain fructans are not allowed on the Elimination Phase of your diet, nor are vegetables which contain more than a minimal amount of polyols. A few vegetables have fructose in excess of glucose. The following vegetables are allowed, because they contain only small amounts of galactans/GOS or short-chain fructans; they do not contain excess fructose; they contain little or no polyols. Vegetable shown in boldface type should be limited to the portion size shown. Serving sizes are suggestions.

Bamboo shoots, ½ C.
Bean sprouts, ½ C.
**Bok choy, ½ C.**
Carrots, 1 medium or ½ C. baby
Celery, 1 medium stalk
Cherry tomatoes, 8 or about 1 C.
Chili pepper, red, 1 small
Chives, green part only, ½ C.
Cucumber, ½ C.
Eggplant, ½ C.
**Fennel bulb, ½ C.**
Globe artichoke or artichoke hearts, ½ C.
**Green bell pepper, ½ C.**
**Green beans, ½ C.**
**Green peas, fresh or frozen, , ½ C.**
Leaf lettuce, 2 C. shredded
**Okra, ½ C.**
Pickle, dill or sour, 1 large
Radishes, 10 small
Red bell pepper, ½ C.
Scallions/green onions, green part only, ½ C.
Spinach, cooked, ½ C.
Spinach, raw, 2 C.
Summer squash, ½ C.
**Sweet potato, ½ C**
Tomatoes, canned without tomato paste or concentrate, ½ C.
Tomatoes, fresh, 1 medium or ½ C.
**Turnip/swede/rutabaga, ½ C.**
Winter squash/pumpkin (AU), ½ C.
Zucchini, ½ C.

*Cooking Tips:*

- Leafy herbs, fresh or dried, such as oregano, basil, parsley, thyme, and rosemary, are allowed.
- It is OK to sauté large pieces of onion or garlic in oil and then remove before consuming. Because fructans are water soluble, onions and garlic should not be cooked in broths or soups.

*Please read labels carefully and avoid the following:*

- Onion powder/dehydrated onion (check packets, mixes, prepared foods of all kinds)
- Garlic powder/dehydrated garlic (check packets, mixes, prepared foods of all kinds)
- Tomato paste (check canned tomatoes, sauces, condiments, pizzas)
- Fructose, crystalline fructose, or high-fructose corn syrup (check sauces, condiments, deli-prepared salads)
- Dehydrated vegetables in whole-food type supplements, including garlic tablets or capsules

*Answer to the following question is on page 111.*

*Q. Where are avocado, beets, broccoli, Brussels sprouts, corn, fennel and pumpkin? They are allowed by some other resources.*

### Allowed Fats

Nuts, seeds and olives are included in this group, because their primary contribution to the diet is fat. Because nuts and seeds do contain small amounts of FODMAPs, only limited portions sizes (boldface type) are allowed. Oils from plant foods do not have any FODMAPs in them.

Milk-based fats usually contain lactose. Small serving sizes (boldface type), with 1 gram or less of lactose per serving, are allowed on the Elimination Phase of your diet. Serving sizes for other fats are suggestions.

**Nuts, any kind except pistachios, ½ oz. or 2 T.**
**Peanut or almond butter, 2 T.**
**Seeds: sesame, pine nuts, sunflower or pumpkin/pepitas, 2 T.**
Coconut meat or flour, 2T.
Oil, any type, including soybean, coconut and garlic-infused, 1 t.
Margarine, 1 t.
Mayonnaise, regular, 1 T.
Tahini, 2 T.
Tartar sauce, 1 T.
Olives, 9 large
Coconut cream, 2 T.
Coconut milk, ¼ C.
Butter, 1 t.
**Cream cheese, 2 T.**
**Half-and-half, 2 T.**
**Heavy cream, whipped, ¼ C.**
**Sour cream, 2 T.**
**Sour cream, low-fat, 2 T.**

*Please read labels carefully and avoid the following:*

- Inulin (check spreads, dressings, sauces, non-dairy toppings or creamers, low-fat sour cream and cream cheese)
- Fructose, crystalline fructose or high-fructose corn syrup (check peanut butter, mayonnaise, non-dairy toppings or creamers)
- Fructo-oligosaccharides/FOS (check non-dairy toppings)
- Onion powder/dehydrated onion (check salad dressings, sauces and condiments)
- Garlic powder/dehydrated garlic (check salad dressings, sauces and condiments)

*Answer to the following question is on page 112.*

*Q. Why are peanuts allowed? Aren't they a legume?*

## Allowed Meats/Milk

Protein is the major dietary contribution of foods in this group, including meat, fish, poultry, milk, and milk products. Note there are no beans, dried peas or lentils allowed as protein sources on the Elimination Phase of your diet, because they contain large amounts of galactans/GOS.

Some dairy products contain large amounts of lactose and are not allowed on the Elimination Phase. Because lactose-free milk and milk products have been specially treated before packaging and are 100% lactose-free, they are allowed in this phase. Lactose-free milk, yogurt, and kefir are encouraged as sources of protein, calcium, and other nutrients. Milk-based foods allowed on the Elimination Phase contain 1 gram of lactose or less per serving. Limit serving sizes if food is shown in boldface type.

Meat, fish, and poultry without added ingredients do not contain FODMAPs. Serving sizes for those items are suggestions.

Beef, 3 oz.
Chicken, 3 oz.
Fish, any kind, 3 oz.
Lamb, 3 oz.
Pork, 3 oz.
Turkey, 3 oz.
Seafood, any kind, 3 oz.
Dry curd cottage cheese, ¼ C.
Cheese, hard, regular or reduced-fat including cheddar, Swiss,
    parmesan, brie, mozzarella, feta, 1 oz.
Cottage cheese, lactose-free, ½ C.
**Goat cheese/chevre, 1 oz.**
**Ricotta cheese, regular, ⅓ C.**
Ricotta cheese, lactose-free, ½ C.
Egg substitute, ½ C.
Egg whites, 4 large
Egg, whole, 1 large
Kefir, lactose-free, 8 fl. oz.
**Kefir, regular, 4 fl. oz.**
Milk, lactose-free, skim or low-fat, 8 fl. oz.
Yogurt, lactose-free, 1 C.
Tofu, 3 oz.

*Please read labels carefully and avoid the following:*

- Beans, including baked beans, kidney, pinto, black, edamame, lima, butter, navy, garbanzo/chickpeas, or any other dried beans, black-eyed peas or any other dried peas (check soups, dips such as hummus, frozen meals, salads)
- Soy beans or soy products such as edamame, soy nuts, soy milk, and tempeh (check vegetarian convenience foods, beverages).
- Lentils, including brown, yellow, and red (check soups, dal)
- Milk (unless it is pre-treated with lactase), nonfat dry milk powder, buttermilk or buttermilk solids
- Whey protein concentrate (unless stated lactose-free)
- Yogurt or yogurt solids (unless stated lactose-free)
- Onion powder/dehydrated onion (check soups, broths, sauces)
- Garlic powder/dehydrated garlic (check soups, broths, sauces)

*These ingredients and descriptions are allowed:*

- Foods "processed in a facility that also makes products containing milk"
- Whey protein isolate
- Soybean lecithin
- Soybean oil
- Guar gum
- Carageenan

Label reading tip for natural cheeses with no added ingredients:

- You can be sure the cheese is lactose-free by verifying the Nutrition Facts panel lists zero grams of sugar per serving.

*Answers to the following questions begin on page 112.*

*Q. I'm lactose-intolerant, so I don't eat any dairy. Plus, I've always read people with IBS should avoid dairy. Are you sure I should be eating these foods?*

*Q. You say that most cheeses and lactose-free milk are OK, but I have had them in the past and I know I felt bad. What could be going on?*

*Q. What does lactose-free milk taste like?*

*Q. I'm lactose-intolerant, but I eat yogurt because they say it is easier to digest. Is that a mistake?*

*Q. I am not lactose-intolerant. Do I still have to use lactose-free milk products?*

*Q. Why isn't goat's milk allowed? I've read it is better for people with GI problems.*

**Allowed Extras**

Even allowed sweets must be limited in quantity on the Elimination Phase, with a maximum of 40 grams of total sugar per serving; don't exceed the portion size shown for the boldface items. Some sweets contain polyols and are not allowed. Some sweets contain excess fructose and are not allowed. Sweets made with wheat, spelt, kamut, or chick pea flower contain fructans and are not allowed. The following foods are allowed in the quantities indicated:

Almond milk, 8 fl. oz.
**Beer, 12 fl. oz.**
Black pepper
**Candy/chocolate made with allowed ingredients, 1 oz.**
Coconut water, 8 fl.oz.
**Coffee, black, brewed, 8 fl. oz., limit one per day**
**Corn syrup (not high-fructose), 1 ½ T.**
**Evaporated cane juice, 1 ½ T.**
**Ice cream, lactose-free, ½ C.**
**Jam or jelly, 1 ½ T.**
**Maple syrup, 100% pure (not "pancake" syrup), 1 ½ T.**
Rice milk, 8 fl. oz.
**Sorbet with allowed ingredients, ½ C.**
**Spirits, 1 fl. oz.**
**Sucrose-sweetened soft drink, 12 fl. oz.**
**Sugar: brown, cane, confectioner's, granulated, 1 ½ T.**
**Spirits, 1 ½ oz.**
**Syrup: cane, sugar, golden, 1 ½ T.**
Tea: black, green, ginger, peppermint, chamomile, brewed, 8 fl. oz.
**Wine, red or white, 4 fl. oz.**

*Please read labels* carefully and avoid the following:

- Honey
- Fructose, crystalline fructose, or high-fructose corn syrup (check soft drinks/soda pop and other beverages, fizzy drink mixes such as Emergen-C®, pancake syrup)
- Molasses (check gums, candies, beverages, energy or snack bars, cookies)
- Spelt, kamut, enriched, bleached, white or wheat flour in any form (check cakes, cookies, muffins, pastries)
- Rosé wine, sweet alcoholic drinks such as margaritas, piña coladas, sweet martinis, sours, and tropicals

- Ice cream (unless stated lactose-free)
- Sorbitol, polydextrose, mannitol, isomalt, xylitol, maltitol, lactitol, or hydrogenated starch hydrolysates (check liquid medications, flavored seltzer water and other beverages, gum, candy, cough drops, frozen desserts, low-carb nutrition and supplement bars, wasabi paste)
- Inulin (check fiber, nutrition or energy bars, frozen desserts)
- Chicory or chicory root (check herbal teas, coffee substitutes, fiber, nutrition or energy bars, frozen desserts)
- Fructo-oligosaccharides/FOS (check low-fat cookies, granola bars, energy bars)
- Polydextrose (check candy, cake, pudding, gelatin desserts, frozen desserts)
- High-fructose corn syrup (check seasoned vinegars, baked goods, syrups, candies, ice creams, sorbets)

*Answers to the following questions begin on page 115.*

*Q. Coffee has FODMAPs? How can that be? Please elaborate.*

*Q. What about herbs, spices, and other flavorings?*

*Q. I'm confused about soy. Is it allowed or isn't it?*

*Q. Can you go into a little more detail about vinegar? I've read some vinegars are bad for people with GI problems and that unfiltered apple cider vinegar is the best; that's the opposite of what you are saying.*

*Q. I keep seeing ads on TV that say high-fructose corn syrup is no different from regular sugar, so why can't I have it on this diet?*

## Summary of Label Reading Tips

**These ingredients are allowed.** Please note that this list is meant to help with label reading. The preceding pages list the grains, starches, fruits, vegetables, fats, meats, milk products and other extras that are allowed.

Aspartame
Baker's yeast
Baking powder
Baking soda/sodium
   bicarbonate
Bar sugar
Beet sugar
Berry sugar
Black pepper
Brown sugar
Cane juice crystals
Cane sugar
Cane syrup
Carageenan
Castor sugar
Chocolate
Cocoa powder
Confectioner's sugar
Corn starch
Corn syrup (not high-
   fructose)
Corn syrup solids
Cultured corn syrup
Dehydrated sugar cane juice
Demerara sugar
Dextrose
Glucose
Granulated sugar
Guar gum
High-maltose corn syrup
Icing sugar
Invert sugar
Malt extract
Maltodextrin
Maltose
Modified food starch
Organic sugar

Pectin
Raw sugar
Refined sugar
Resistant starch
Saccharine
Salt
Soy lecithin
Soy sauce
Soybean oil
Stevia
Sucrose
Sugar syrup
Superfine sugar
Sucralose
Vinegar
Vital wheat gluten
Wheat starch
Whey protein isolate
Xanthan gum

**These ingredients are NOT allowed.** Please note that this list is meant to help with label reading and is not an exhaustive list of items that are "not allowed." As a rule, any food not specifically named on the "allowed" lists should not be eaten during the Elimination Phase of the diet

Agave syrup
All-purpose flour
Bulgur wheat
Brown rice syrup
Chicory root extract
Crystalline fructose
Dry milk solids
Enriched flour
Fructo-oligosaccharides/FOS
Fructose
Fructose solids
Fruit juice concentrates (any type)
Glycerin
Goat's milk (unless lactose-free)
High-fructose corn syrup (HFCS)
Honey
Hydrogenated starch hydrolysates
Inulin
Isomalt
Kamut
Lactitol
Lactulose
Maltitol
Mannitol
Miso
Molasses
Polydextrose
Sorbitol
Spelt
Sprouted wheat
Texturized vegetable protein
Tomato paste
Wheat berries
Whey protein concentrate (unless lactose-free)
White flour
Whole wheat flour
Xylitol

*Answers to the following questions begin on page 118.*

*Q. I am on the go all the time and usually eat a lot of pre-packaged fiber, fruit, protein or snack bars. What can I do now?*

*Q. Why isn't agave syrup allowed? It's supposed to be all natural and better for your blood sugar.*

*Q. I can't believe gluten is allowed on this diet. Isn't that bad for people with gut problems? How can I trust the rest of your advice you if you allow gluten?*

*Q. How can I evaluate the information on the Nutrition Facts panel to figure out whether I can eat a food?*

*Q. One of my medications contains glycerin, lactose, or another ingredient that is "not allowed." What should I do?*

*Q. What should I look for in a multi-vitamin with minerals supplement?*

## Beyond the Allowed Food Lists

There are thousands of foods in the world that do not appear on the "allowed" food lists in this book. Some of them are specifically "not allowed" until the Challenge Phase of the diet. What about the many foods, beverages, and ingredients that are not mentioned at all? They are not mentioned because I was unable to find published material about their nutrient composition. Therefore, I couldn't say for sure whether they were allowed or not allowed.

Happily, this has the effect of keeping the FODMAP Elimination Diet rather simple. It certainly doesn't mean that foods not mentioned in the book are off limits for you. Not at all; just avoid them during the Elimination and Challenge Phases of the FODMAP Elimination Diet. After the Challenge Phase of the diet is over, feel free to resume other foods that you tolerated in the past. You will find out soon enough if they cause your IBS symptoms to return.

## Step 5: Monitor your symptoms and compare them to baseline.

*"Did my symptoms go away? Oh yes, they did! It was a dramatic difference, just like night and day. It was like going back to a state of well-being I had left long ago and forgot existed."—C.C.*

After you have been on the Elimination Phase of the diet for approximately two weeks, return to your Symptom Worksheet. Record your current symptoms and their effects on your life. If the FODMAP Elimination Phase has done its job, you may be feeling so much better by now that you don't need any worksheets or numbers to tell you so. If your results have been less dramatic, the worksheet will be especially helpful.

Let us recap how you will know whether the diet is working. Review your records and compare the symptoms you were experiencing at the baseline (before the diet) to the symptoms you experienced during the first week of the diet. If the Elimination Diet is working, there should be a noticeable drop in both the number and type of symptoms you are experiencing and the negative impact they are having on your life. The extent to which you benefit from the diet is ultimately a judgment call, using these numbers as a guide. You are the one who decides whether eliminating FODMAP carbohydrates significantly improves your symptoms. You will come to one of two tentative conclusions:

## Your Symptoms Have Improved Dramatically

If you decide that your symptoms have improved markedly, you can move on to the Challenge Phase of the FODMAP Elimination Diet whenever you are ready.

## Your Symptoms Have Not Improved or Have Improved Just a Little

If you follow this diet faithfully and carefully and you are still no better after one two weeks, it might be helpful to write down everything you eat and drink for a few days. Ask someone else to review the diet record with you and compare it to the allowed food lists, looking for unintentional sources of FODMAPs in your food.

Ask yourself whether you have been making exceptions for any reason. Don't worry, there is no shame in this—we have all experienced situations where we are not in control of the food and have to eat what is served. Unfortunately, exceptions can ruin your experiment. If you find your diet wasn't as FODMAP friendly as you had hoped, you may wish to continue the Elimination Phase for another week or two.

You may be aware of other possible factors that held back potential improvement in your symptoms, such as a particularly stressful week or a viral illness. If that is the case, continue the Elimination Phase for another week and reassess.

There is also the chance that you may be at the extreme end of intolerance for FODMAPs. For one additional week, eliminate all foods in **bold** type, since they do contain small amounts. Do this for only one week, as an experiment. I do not encourage anyone to permanently stop eating fruits, low-lactose milk products, nuts or any other large group of foods unless there is a very good reason. At the end of that third week, if there is still no improvement, there is probably little to be gained by continuing. Please return to your regular diet and talk to your dietitian or doctor for guidance about other treatment options.

*Answers to the following questions begin on page 121.*

*Q. I have lost some weight while on the Elimination Phase of the diet. Is that OK?*

*Q. I am working with a dietitian. When is the best time to schedule a follow up appointment?*

*Q. The Elimination Phase is working a little too well! Even though I have diarrhea-predominant IBS, I am actually feeling a little constipated. What should I do?*

Part 1: The Program    57

# Chapter 2: The Challenge Phase

## Step 6: Reintroduce FODMAPs in a series of controlled challenges; monitor symptoms.

During the Challenge Phase of the elimination diet, you will actually be trying to provoke your IBS symptoms, so that you can learn more specifically which types of FODMAPs are problems for you. This information will help you figure out how to eat going forward. I want to emphasize that you will learn the most if you approach the Challenge Phase with as much discipline as you can muster. If you start adding things back to your diet willy-nilly, you will be just as confused in a month as you were before you started.

It will take approximately six weeks to work your way through the Challenge Phase of the diet. After that, the process of experimenting with new foods can continue in a more informal way.

Because IBS symptoms may result from a challenge, be sure to plan the challenge for a time when you can afford to feel unwell for a day or two.

### Directions for the Challenge Phase

Use the Challenge Phase Worksheet, below, to keep track of what you eat during each challenge and what the results are. The worksheet can also be downloaded from www.ibsfree.net.

- Continue to eat all the foods normally allowed on the basic elimination diet in addition to the "challenge" foods
- Do only one challenge at a time. Don't add challenges on top of each other.
- It is important to challenge only one type of FODMAP at a time, to avoid becoming confused about the cause of symptoms. Keep your eye on the ball and don't let FODMAPs drift back into your diet during the Challenge Phase. Make sure the foods you challenge with don't contain other FODMAPs—for example, when doing a lactose challenge, choose plain or vanilla yogurt that does not contain honey, high-fructose corn syrup, inulin, fruit juice concentrate, or any other type of FODMAP.
- The items toward the bottom of each challenge food list contain the least of the targeted FODMAP and won't be as useful for the challenge. For example, your challenge won't

have as much punch if you use soy milk instead of baked beans for your galactans/GOS challenge.

- The first day of each challenge, be cautious and have only a small portion of food containing the targeted FODMAP. For example, on the first day of the fructans challenge, have just one piece of bread. This is to protect you from the possibility of a severe reaction you might get with a large portion if you are extremely intolerant to one of the FODMAPs.

- If you feel unwell after the cautious challenge, do not proceed. Return to the elimination diet and try the cautious challenge again some other time.

- On the second day, give yourself a bigger challenge. Do not be tentative about it. You are trying to provoke symptoms. Eat the largest portions from the test group that might be typical for you. For example, on the second day of the fructans challenge, have a bagel for breakfast, a big sandwich for lunch, plain cake, cookies, or crackers for snacks, and a plate of whole wheat spaghetti with lots of onions and garlic for dinner.

- Since you will only be challenging with one type of FODMAP carbohydrate at a time, you will have to eat quite a bit of it to get the total FODMAPs load you may have had from the combination of foods you were eating before. However, don't overdo polyols or galactans/GOS. Don't eat more than one or two sugar-free, polyol-sweetened candies unless you had been accustomed to doing so in the past.

- You can stop before the end of the day if you are experiencing painful symptoms.

- Always allow at least three days on the basic elimination diet between each challenge, longer if you suffer from constipation or if the Challenge Phase provoked severe symptoms.

- When you are ready, select and carry out the next challenge.

- The order of the challenges doesn't matter. Do the one that is the most important to you first and leave the foods you can easily do without for last. If you can't decide which one to do first, begin with the lactose challenge; it is the easiest one to plan and interpret.

**Challenge Phase Worksheet**

*Lactose Challenge*

Day 1: Cautious Challenge. I ate/drank:


Day 2: Full Challenge. I ate/drank:


My results:



*Fructose Challenge*

Day 1: Cautious Fructose


Day 2: Full Fructose Part A Challenge. I ate/drank:


Day 3: Add Fructose Part B Challenge foods. I ate/drank:


My results:

## *Fructans Challenge*

Day 1: Cautious Challenge. I ate:


Day 2: Full Challenge. I ate:


My results:


## *Polyols Challenge*

Day 1 Cautious Challenge: I ate/drank:


Day 2: Full Challenge. I ate/drank:


My results:


## *Galactans/GOS Challenge*

Day 1 Cautious Challenge: I ate/drank:


Day 2: Full Challenge. I ate/drank:


My results:

**Lactose Challenge**

Foods toward the top of the list contain more lactose per serving and will be more effective during the challenge than foods lower on the list. None of the milk products used during the lactose challenge should be lactose-free. Do not take lactase tablets with the food. Check labels to make sure that they do not contain honey, high-fructose corn syrup, inulin, or other FODMAPs. Foods to use during your lactose challenge:

Evaporated milk
Yogurt with added whey, whey concentrate, or nonfat-dry milk, plain or sweetened with sugar only
Fluid milk, whole, low-fat or non-fat
Eggnog
Goat's milk
Milkshake, vanilla or strawberry
Frozen yogurt, ice milk, or soft-serve ice cream, vanilla or strawberry
Regular yogurt, plain or sweetened with sugar only
Greek yogurt, plain or sweetened with sugar only
Premium, full-fat ice cream, sweetened with sugar only
Cottage cheese, whole, low-fat or non-fat
Kefir, plain or sweetened with sugar only

*Answers to the following questions begin on page 122.*

*Q. Where did you get the data used to rank the lactose content of these foods?*

*Q. Is there a way to distinguish lactose intolerance from casein sensitivity during the Challenge Phase?*

*Q. I already know I am lactose-intolerant—do I have to do that challenge?*

**Fructose Challenge—Part A**

Foods toward the top of the list contain more fructose in excess of glucose per serving and will be more effective during the challenge than foods lower on the list. Remember to check ingredients and omit foods that contain other sources of FODMAPs. HFCS=high-fructose corn syrup. Foods to use during your fructose challenge:

Beverages with crystalline fructose, such as Glaceau Vitamin Water®, Emergen-C® Fizzy Drink Mix
Agave syrup or nectar
Carbonated soft drink, iced tea, or punch with HFCS, especially bottled Pepsi®, Coke® and Sprite®
Barbecue sauce with HFCS
Pancake syrup with HFCS
Ketchup with HFCS
Jam or jelly with HFCS
Honey
Fruits and juices, allowed, larger servings
Fruits, allowed, dried, such as raisins and dried cranberries
Fruit juice concentrate or fruit leathers made from allowed fruits
Mango, fresh or dried
Asparagus
Molasses

### Fructose Challenge—Part B

Fruits toward the top of this list have more fructose in excess of glucose and more polyols per serving and will be more effective during the challenge than foods lower on the list. Continue your fructose challenge by adding these items on the third day.

Fruit juice concentrate (pear, apple)
Fruit leathers (pear, peach, apple)
Pears and pear juice
Peaches
Watermelon
Apples and apple juice
Apple cider
Apple sauce

**Fructans Challenge**

Foods toward the top of the list contain more fructans per serving and will be more effective during the challenge than foods lower on the list. Remember to check ingredients and omit other foods high in FODMAPs. "Yeast breads or baked goods" include bread, bagels, English muffins, pizza crust, flour tortillas, rolls, cookies, cakes, muffins, pastries, pretzels, and crackers. Foods to use during your fructans challenge:

Fiber, protein, or snack bars with chicory root extract or inulin
High-fiber breakfast cereals with chicory root, inulin, wheat bran,
     rye, or barley
Yeast breads or baked goods made with rye
Wheat berries or bulgur wheat
Barley
Couscous
Gnocchi
Broccoli*
Onions, onion powder
Radicchio
Brussels sprouts*
Cabbage*
Kale
Beets/beetroot
Nuts, pecans or walnuts, bigger/more servings
Seeds, sesame or pine nuts, bigger/more servings
Shallots
Scallions (white part)
Garlic, garlic powder
Pasta, white or whole wheat
Yeast breads or baked goods made with white, whole wheat, or
     multigrain flour
Yeast breads or baked goods made with spelt flour
Sourdough (no added yeast) white or wheat bread
Sourdough (no added yeast) spelt bread
Larger portions of allowed, boldface vegetables

* Also contains polyols

*Answers to the following questions begin on page 122.*

*Q. The ranking order of the foods in the fructans category seems off. I've read that garlic has more fructans than any other food, but you've ranked it toward the bottom of the list. What gives?*

*Q. Why is sourdough bread listed lower than other breads?*

*Q .If I react badly to wheat products, is there a way to distinguish non-celiac gluten intolerance from fructans intolerance during the Challenge Phase?*

*Q. I was fine when I challenged with fructans. What's the harm in eating bread while I do the rest of the challenges?*

## Polyols Challenge

Foods toward the top of the list contain more polyols per serving and will be more effective during the challenge than foods lower on the list. Foods and ingredients to use during your polyols challenge:

Candy or cough drops, "sugar-free" with maltitol, sorbitol, isomalt, lactitol, mannitol, xylitol, polydextrose, or hydrogenated starch hydrolysates. Use caution, as some are very high in polyols
Low-carb bars
Prune juice
Prunes
Figs, dried
Blackberries
Mushrooms, all kinds
Cauliflower
Dates
Sweet cherries
Pumpkin (U.S.)
Gum, "sugar-free" with maltitol, sorbitol, isomalt, lactitol, mannitol, xylitol, polydextrose, or hydrogenated starch hydrolysates
Snow peas, sugar snap peas*
Peaches
Nectarines
Apricots
Avocado
Plums
Fennel leaves
Sweet corn, fresh, frozen, canned
Figs, fresh

*Also contains fructans

**Galactans/GOS Challenge:**

Galactans are also known as galacto-oligosaccharides (GOS). Foods toward the top of the list have more galactans/GOS per serving and will be more effective during the challenge than foods lower on the list. Foods to use during your galactans challenge:

Dried/split peas*
Dried/canned beans*
Lentils
Butter/lima beans
Pistachios*
Chickpeas or hummus
Tempeh
Veggie-burgers, soy
Soy milk
Sunflower seeds, bigger/more servings
Almonds, bigger/more servings
Coffee, bigger/more servings

* Also contain significant fructans

## Step 7: Evaluate your results and modify your diet accordingly.

You've worked hard to eliminate FODMAPs from your diet, and you have completed your food challenges. You kept close track of your symptoms during the challenges, and you now have an idea which categories of FODMAPs are symptom triggers for you. At this point, if you are like most of my clients, you are still left with a number of questions about how to eat from here on. This section is a bit tricky, because each and every one of you will have had a unique experience on this diet and will have to work out your own combination of meal planning strategies.

The general idea is that by juggling your food intake so the overall FODMAP burden of the meal or day stays within your personal limits, you can manage your symptoms. The following questions address specific situations you may have encountered during the Challenge Phase. The answers will help you cope with your problem FODMAPs, so that you don't have to give up eating your favorite foods altogether. Read the answers to questions that interest you.

*Answers to the following questions begin on page 124.*

*Q. How long does it take for symptoms to appear after eating an offending food? What is the significance of the timing?*

*Q. I ate one piece of bread for my "cautious" fructans challenge. Boy, was I sick! What should I do next?*

*Q. I challenged a particular group of FODMAPs and I had no symptoms. Can I go back to eating them now?*

*Q. I challenged a particular group of FODMAPs and my symptoms were severe. How can I cope with that?*

*Q. I was kind of uncomfortable during one of the challenges, but it really wasn't too bad. Should I re-challenge it?*

*Q. If I react badly to one food within a group, should I assume that I can't tolerate all the other foods in that group. For example, if I can't tolerate bread, does that mean I need to avoid all the foods in the fructan group?*

*Q. I feel a lot better, but I still have some gas. How can I get rid of it?*

*Q. The diet didn't work for me at all. What can I take away from this experience?*

*Q. Friday pizza night with the family is very important to me and I don't want to give it up, even though too many fructans make me feel crummy. How can I manage this?*

*Q. Since I've been on this diet, it seems like I am having a problem with a particular food that isn't even high in FODMAPs. Why am I noticing this now?*

*Q. Are there any absolutely prohibited foods after the Challenge Phase?*

*Q. What if I fail all the FODMAP challenges?*

*Q. Will my FODMAP intolerance ever get better, or am I stuck with this problem for life?*

*Q. It appears I am lactose-intolerant. Should I just quit drinking milk?*

*Q. I've heard that some medications contain lactose. If I'm lactose-intolerant, what should I do about this?*

*Q. Fructose was the worst one for me. Is there anything equivalent to lactase tablets that will help me digest fructose?*

*Q. I have trouble with fructans. Any special tips for me?*

*Q. What about an enzyme to break down fructans?*

*Q. Can I work around the fructans problem by eating gluten-free bread and pizza dough?*

*Q. If I have fructose malabsorption, do I automatically have to limit fructans as well, since fructans are chains of fructose molecules linked together?*

*Q. Those polyols killed me. Is there any help for that?*

*Q. Are there any specific tips for people who don't tolerate galactans/GOS?*

*Q. I don't eat meat. How should I manage that, given the high-FODMAP content of legumes (pulses), which I rely on for protein?*

*Q. I am looking at a food label and everything looks OK except for that one joy-killer there toward the end of the ingredients list. Can I eat this food?*

*Q. What are probiotics and should I take them?*

## Step 8: Enjoy the most liberal and varied diet you can tolerate without triggering your symptoms.

That's it, the final step in the process. Each word in that sentence is important. I hope that you will be able to *enjoy* foods that make you feel good, not have to fear food or eating. Don't over-restrict yourself based on faulty or outdated assumptions. *Liberalize* your diet as much as possible by testing foods out for yourself. *Variety* in the diet is important to make sure you get a full range of nutrients. Even if you have to stick pretty close to the Elimination Phase in the long term, choose as much variety as you can from each food list. Try to eat as much fiber as *you* can tolerate. *You* are the judge of what foods are right for your IBS; you needn't be obliged to eliminate any food or food group just on principle. Your *symptoms* will be your guide.

# Chapter 3: Alternate Approach

There may be times when it is appropriate to take the opposite approach to the elimination diet. As you know, I usually recommend eliminating all the FODMAPs at the beginning, then adding them back one by one to see what happens. This section describes another approach: *removing* the FODMAPs one by one, while keeping the rest of the usual diet intact.

The main reason I prefer the first approach is for its dramatic effect. My clients, understandably, want to feel better immediately. They have played around with ineffective diets for years and are impatient for results. They want to know within a week or two whether the FODMAP Elimination Diet holds the answers for them.

However, removing FODMAPs one group at a time might be a better choice if you already have a lot of other dietary limitations or are not very flexible in your food preferences (picky eaters, you know who you are). It may be a better choice for children or young teenagers, when parents or health providers do not think it physically or emotionally wise to make diet change too much of a production. Also, it may be more practical for someone who does not have much control over menu and food preparation, for example, an elderly person in an assisted living facility or nursing home.

If you want to take this alternate approach, where should you begin? The following worksheet will help. You can use it to figure out which types of FODMAPs are most prominent in your diet. This worksheet is not a scientifically validated screening tool; it is based on common sense. The foods you eat most often have a bigger influence on your health than the ones you eat once in a while. Also, you may be blind to your trigger foods like bread and pasta because you were always told they were safe for IBS. You may be deliberately eating some FODMAP-containing foods, such as apples and pears, for their health benefits, without realizing they are causing you digestive distress. You must discover which types of carbohydrates are right for *you*.

The worksheet can be downloaded from www.ibsfree.net.

## FODMAP Frequency Worksheet

For each of the following foods, calculate and write down the number of serving or units per week you eat of that food in the space provided. Do your best to add up your total intake for a typical seven-day week. If you have difficulty with these calculations, read the examples carefully and see if one of them can help you.

The serving size for many foods is described in terms of cups (C.) or tablespoons (T.); for example, cottage cheese, ½ C. You probably don't usually measure your cottage cheese before you eat it! Before you complete this questionnaire, get out some measuring cups and measuring spoons and remind yourself what ½ cup, 1 cup, 1 tablespoon and 1 teaspoon of food look like. Remember, measure the amount of food in the measuring cups and spoons level with the top, not "heaping." Measure some foods into your usual plates, bowls and cups. This brief exercise should prepare you to complete this worksheet more accurately.

If the serving size for the food is described in terms of ounces (oz.) or pounds (lbs.), you don't have to actually weigh the food. You may get the information you need from the food label. One way to do this is to compare the weight of the whole package to the amount you eat in a week. Another way is to check the Nutrition Facts panel on the packaging. At the top of the panel you will usually find the serving size and weight in grams. If you are actually eating more than the listed serving size, be sure to take that into account. Thirty grams is roughly equal to 1 ounce.

*Example 1*: You eat pizza every Friday night. You eat 4 slices of pizza at that meal. The unit indicated for pizza is "½ slice." You are eating eight "½ slices" per week. You would write "8" in the space provided.

*Example 2*: You eat 3 sandwiches per week on wraps. There are 8 wraps in a 16-oz.package, therefore, each of your wraps weighs 2 oz. The unit indicated for wraps is "1 oz." Each of your wraps is equal to two "1 oz." portions, so you would write "6" in the space provided.

*Example 3*: You eat one very large cookie a week from the canteen at work. At your request, the cafeteria worker checks the frozen dough package for you and tells you the cookie weighs 3 oz. The unit for cookies is "1 oz."; your cookie is equal to 3 "1 oz." cookies, so you would write "3" in the space provided.

*Example 5*: You go through a 1 lb. loaf of bread each week. There are 16 oz. in 1 lb., so you would write "16" in the space provided.

*Example 6*: The package of Fiber One cereal you eat seven days a week says the serving size is 1 cup. You check your portion and find you are serving yourself 2 cups. Therefore, in seven days you are eating 14 servings, so you would write "14" in the space provided.

Note, there may be certain foods you eat only in season; write "0" for the number of servings of out-of-season foods, since you are not currently eating them. Or, if you are known to eat large portions of these foods when they *are* in season, you could put a star in the blank space for emphasis.

## Lactose Group

_____Evaporated milk, 8 fl. oz. or 1 C.

_____Yogurt with added whey, whey concentrate or nonfat dry milk, plain or sweetened with sugar only, 1 C.

_____Fluid milk, 8 fl. oz. or 1 C.

_____Eggnog, 8 fl. oz. or 1 C.

_____Goat's milk, 8 fl. oz. or 1 C.

_____Milkshake, 8 fl. oz. or 1 C.

_____Ice cream, frozen yogurt, ice milk, or soft-serve ice cream, 1 C.

_____Regular yogurt, 1 C.

_____Greek yogurt, 1 C.

_____Cottage cheese, ½ C

_____Kefir, 8 fl. oz. or 1 C.

_____Whey concentrate protein powder, 1 scoop

## Fructose Group

*HFCS=High Fructose Corn Syrup*

_____Beverages with crystalline fructose, such as Glaceau Vitamin Water®, Emergen-C® fizzy drink mix, 8 fl. oz. or 1 C.

_____Carbonated soft drink, iced tea or punch with HFCS, such as Pepsi®, Coke®, Sprite®, juice "cocktails," 8 fl. oz. or 1 C.

_____Agave syrup or nectar, 2T.

_____Barbecue sauce with HFCS, 2T.

_____Pancake syrup with HFCS, 2 T.

_____Jam or jelly with HFCS, 2T.

_____Honey, 2T.

_____Molasses, 2T.

_____Gummy or chewable multivitamin supplements with fructose, 1 dose (check nutrition info for size of dose)

_____Pears, 1 medium

_____Apples, 1 medium

_____Other fruit, whole, 1 medium

_____Fruit, cut up, fresh, canned or frozen, ½ C.

_____Fruit juice, 4 fl. oz. or ½ C.

_____Dried fruit or trail mix with fruit, including raisins, dried cranberries, prunes, apricots, dates, figs, ¼ C.

_____Fruit leathers, 1 piece

## Fructans Group

_____Fiber, protein, or snack bars with chicory root extract or inulin, 1 bar

_____High-fiber breakfast cereals with chicory root, inulin, wheat bran, rye, barley, 1 serving (check nutrition info for the serving size—if your portion is bigger, count multiple servings)

_____Yeast breads or baked goods made with rye, 1 oz.

_____Barley, ½ C. cooked

_____Bulgur wheat, ½ C. cooked

_____Couscous, ½ C. cooked

_____Gnocchi, 1 C.

_____Beet/beetroot, ½ C.  cooked

_____Broccoli, ½ C.

_____Brussels sprouts, ½ C.

_____Onions, raw ½ C. or ¼ C. cooked

_____Scallions (white part), ½ C.

_____Garlic, 1 clove or 1 t.

_____Shallots, ¼ C. cooked

_____Pasta, white or whole wheat, ½ C. cooked

_____Radicchio, ½ C.

_____Cabbage, ½ C.

_____Kale, ½ C. cooked

_____Yeast breads, English muffins, rolls tortillas, pitas or chapatis made with white, whole wheat, or multigrain flour, 1 oz.

_____Cookies made with white, whole wheat, or multigrain flour, 1 oz. (1 small or ⅓ large cookie)

_____Cake or muffins made with white, whole wheat, or multigrain flour, ½ fast food serving

_____Donuts, 1

_____Crackers or pretzels made with white, whole wheat, or multigrain flour, 1 oz. or ½ C.

_____Biscuits or scones made with white, whole wheat, or multigrain flour, 1 oz (1 small or ⅓ large)

_____Pizza crust made with white, whole wheat, or multigrain flour, ½ slice

## Polyols Group

_____Candy or cough drops, "sugar-free" with maltitol, sorbitol, isomalt, lactitol, mannitol, xylitol, polydextrose, or hydrogenated starch hydrolysates, 1 serving (check nutrition info for serving size)

_____Liquid medication with maltitol, sorbitol, isomalt, lactitol, mannitol, xylitol, polydextrose, or hydrogenated starch hydrolysates, 1 dose

_____Low-carb bars, 1 serving (check nutrition info for serving size)

Prune juice, 4 fl. oz.

_____Prunes, ¼ C.

_____Figs, dried, ¼ C.

_____Blackberries, ½ C.

_____Mushrooms, ½ C. cooked or 1 C. raw

_____Cauliflower, ½ C.

_____Dates, ¼ C.

_____Sweet Cherries, ½ C.

_____Gum, "sugar free" with maltitol, sorbitol, isomalt, lactitol, mannitol , xylitol, polydextrose, or hydrogenated starch hydrolysates, 1 piece

_____Snow peas, ½ C.

_____Peaches, white or yellow, ½ C.

_____Nectarines, ½ C.

_____Apricots, ½ C. raw or ¼ C. dried

_____Avocado, ½ C.

_____Plum, ½ C.

_____Fennel leaves, ½ C. raw or ½ C. cooked

_____Sweet corn, fresh, frozen, canned, ½ C.

_____Figs, fresh, ½ C.

## Galactans/GOS Group

_____Dried/split peas, ½ C. cooked
_____Dried or canned beans, ½ C. cooked
_____Lentils, ½ C. cooked
_____Butter/lima beans, ½ C. cooked
_____Chick peas or hummus, ½ C. cooked
_____Tempeh, ½ C.
_____Veggie-burgers, soy, 1
_____Soy milk, 8 fl. oz.
_____Coffee, reg. or de-caf., 8 fl. oz.

## Questionnaire Summary

Write in the total servings per week for each of the following food groups:

_____Lactose

_____Fructose

_____Fructans

_____Polyols

_____Galactans/GOS

### Applying the Results of the FODMAP Frequency Worksheet

As you review your food frequency questionnaire summary, you may see a group that clearly emerges as the primary source of FODMAPs in your diet. That is the group you should eliminate first in this alternate approach to the FODMAP Elimination Diet. Before you start, however, please take the time to rate your symptoms using the Symptom Worksheet (download from www.ibsfree.net) to establish a baseline symptom profile. The worksheet will be extremely helpful later for deciding whether elimination of a particular food group makes a difference for you.

Next, select one group of FODMAPs from the food frequency questionnaire to eliminate. For seven days, do not eat any of the foods listed in that section of the questionnaire (important exception—do not stop taking prescribed liquid medications without guidance from the prescribing physician). For example, if you are eliminating the lactose group, for one week do not eat or drink any cottage cheese, milk, yogurt, frozen yogurt, or ice cream. Don't make any exceptions, just for this one week. Monitor your symptoms and record your impressions during the week. If there is a noticeable reduction in your symptoms compared to the baseline week, you may have found an area of your diet that you can modify to keep your symptoms well managed.

Return to your usual diet, including the tested group, for a few days. Do your symptoms return? If so, that is further proof that this part of your diet is responsible, at least in part, for your symptoms. Review Step 7 and Step 8 of the program for tips and techniques on coping with your findings. Consult a registered dietitian if you need additional help modifying your diet.

Work your way through each group, giving yourself a few days in between to return to your usual diet.

# PART 2: THE DETAILS

## *Chapter 4: The Science behind the Diet*

The first section of Part 2 goes into more detail about the physiology, biology and food science of carbohydrate malabsorption and FODMAPs. It is meant for more ambitious lay readers as well as health care providers and may answer some of the questions that are on your mind about the science behind the diet.

The next section of Part 2 contains follow-up questions and answers about the diet that have been submitted to me by readers and colleagues. My objective in pulling these out into Part 2 is to keep Part 1 as simple and streamlined as possible. If you prefer, you can skip the biochemistry and go directly to Chapter 5.

### Understanding Carbohydrate Malabsorption

*What are Carbohydrates?*

Carbohydrates are substances in food that consist of a single sugar molecule or multiples of them in various forms. Along with protein and fat, carbohydrates provide the body with energy. Many foods provide a combination of protein, carbohydrates, and fats. Significant amounts of carbohydrates are found in sweets, sweetened beverages, cereals, grains, fruits, vegetables, and milk products. Few or no carbohydrates are present in meat, fish, poultry, nuts, seeds, fats, or oils.

Sugars are the most basic type of carbohydrate. Monosaccharides consist of just one sugar molecule, all by itself. Glucose, fructose (fruit sugar), and galactose are examples of monosaccharides.

Disaccharides consist of two sugar molecules linked together. Examples include sucrose (granulated sugar) and lactose (milk sugar).

### Three Common Monosaccharides

Fructose          Glucose          Galactose

### Two Common Disaccharides

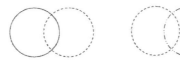

Sucrose = Fructose          Lactose = Glucose
+ Glucose          + Galactose

### An Oligosaccharide (Fructan)

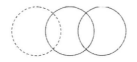

Glucose + Fructose + Fructose

Polyols, or sugar alcohols, are sometimes considered sugars. Examples of polyols are sorbitol, xylitol, and mannitol.

Starches and dietary fiber are examples of complex carbohydrates. Complex carbohydrates are also known as oligosaccharides or polysaccharides, depending on the length and complexity of the sugar chains. Oligosaccharides are short, simple chains of sugars which give easy access to microbes for rapid fermentation, one of the defining criteria for FODMAPs. Polysaccharides have longer chains and more complex structures, with lots of branching and folding. It takes longer for them to be fully fermented by microbes, so they are not FODMAPs.

Starches consist primarily of long, interlocking chains of glucose or fructose units (polysaccharides). Examples of foods containing large amounts of starch are rice, wheat, corn, and potatoes. Most starches can be digested and absorbed by the human body ("modified" or "resistant" starch is less digestible), so they are not FODMAPs.

Dietary fiber consists of non-digestible complex carbohydrates found in plants. Fructans and galactans are dietary fibers. Galactans are sometimes referred to as galacto-oligosaccharides (GOS). Dietary fibers are not broken down by human digestive enzymes. Well-known sources of dietary fiber include whole grains, dried peas and beans, fruits, and vegetables. There are many different systems for naming and categorizing different types of fiber that I will not get into here because they are less relevant to the diets of people with IBS. The main distinction to focus on with regard to FODMAPs is whether or not the fiber is rapidly fermentable. It matters less whether the fiber is soluble or insoluble, unlike the high premium put on soluble fiber by some other approaches to treating IBS. In fact, when it comes to FODMAPs in food, water solubility is a negative. The soluble fibers in onions, garlic, and coffee beans, which are fermentable, can make their way into beverages and soup broths during preparation, and need to be avoided on the Elimination Phase of the FODMAP diet.

### Digestion and Absorption of Carbohydrates

Digestion is the process of breaking food carbohydrates, proteins, and fats down to their smallest units. During digestion, complex carbohydrates are broken down to simple sugars.

Digestion of carbohydrates begins in your mouth. Your teeth chew and grind the food, mixing it with saliva. Saliva contains enzymes that begin the digestive process.

Carbohydrates in your food are further broken down by enzymes in your small intestine. When they are fully digested, they are reduced to their basic units, the monosaccharides glucose, fructose, and galactose. These simple sugars then must pass through the lining of the small intestine into the blood stream, where they are carried off to serve as fuel for your body. This process is called absorption.

There are several interesting details about fructose absorption that help us understand why it is affected by other nutrients consumed at the same meal. It appears there are probably two different ways in which fructose is absorbed through the cell walls of the small intestine. The first is a low-capacity type of diffusion, in which a fructose molecule can pass through the cell wall on its own. Extra fructose is apparently swept along via this mechanism when amino acids are being absorbed at the same time.

The second mechanism is a transport system that only works when there is one glucose molecule available for each fructose molecule. If there are no glucose-fructose pairs, there is no absorption. This explains why granulated sugar, which contains an equal amount of glucose and fructose, is well tolerated in moderation, even by fructose-intolerant individuals. Also, fruits such as berries, certain melons, and citrus fruits, which do not have excess of fructose over glucose, can be tolerated in small servings. However, the fructose- intolerant individual could still experience symptoms if very large portions of these "allowed" foods or beverages are consumed.

### What Is Malabsorption?

If anything prevents carbohydrates from being broken down or passing through the lining of the small intestine, malabsorption is said to occur. There are many possible causes of malabsorption, among them:

- Lack or shortage of the necessary digestive enzymes. This is a common cause of lactose (milk sugar) malabsorption in adults.
- Fast intestinal transit time. Food is catapulted through your system without enough time for digestive enzymes to work or for absorption to occur.
- Total amount of sugar in the meal exceeds the capacity of the small intestine to digest and absorb it. In this situation, fructose or lactose malabsorption should be considered a normal outcome of overindulging.
- Composition of the meal. Fructose is absorbed more completely in the presence of glucose and less completely in the presence of sugar alcohols.
- Damage to the lining of the small intestine  for example, from food poisoning, a virus, untreated celiac disease, or Crohn's disease—might prevent normal enzyme production or absorption.
- Short bowel syndrome. If any length of the small intestine has been surgically removed, malabsorption can occur.
- Some carbohydrates, such as the dietary fibers found in wheat bran or beans, are not meant to be digested or absorbed in the small intestine. Humans do not have the digestive enzymes to break down these dietary fibers.

When carbohydrates are malabsorbed in the small intestine, they pass into the large intestine, where they can cause chaos for individuals with FODMAP-sensitive IBS. If small intestinal bacterial overgrowth (SIBO) is part of the clinical picture, FODMAPs can contribute to symptoms originating in the small intestine, as well.

## Understanding Osmosis

A common characteristic of FODMAPs is their high degree of osmotic activity. Osmosis, in this setting, is the movement of water through the semi-permeable cell membranes of the gut wall, attracted by a higher concentration of sugar inside the lumen of the large intestine.

One of the main functions of your large intestine is to reabsorb water from your stool into your bloodstream, turning stool from a liquid into more of a solid form, ready for excretion. Osmotically active carbohydrates, when malabsorbed, disrupt this process. The resulting watery, urgent bowel movement is sometimes termed osmotic diarrhea.

I wish it were as easy to understand how the osmotically active aspect of FODMAPs intersects with the tendency of some people with IBS to experience constipation, rather than diarrhea. Gut motility is an incredibly complex function. Inputs from the composition of the diet are only one factor affecting transit time, along with hormones, neurotransmitters, inflammation, and gut bacteria. We know that people with constipation tend to be colonized by bacteria that produce methane instead of, or along with, hydrogen. Perhaps the fermentable aspect of FODMAPs has the greater import for folks with constipation, as FODMAPs encourage the activity of methane producing bacteria, which in turn somehow promote constipation. For now, I think it can rightly be said that FODMAPs affect fluid balance in the gut in unpredictable ways. In my practice, I have seen that a low-FODMAP diet is often capable of improving the symptoms of constipation-predominant IBS.

## Understanding Fermentation

FODMAPs share the trait of being rapidly fermentable by the resident bacteria in the gut. Your large intestine is populated by billions of bacteria. In fact, microbes outnumber human cells in your body ten to one! That is normal. Bacteria need energy to survive, and they get it by eating the simple sugars and complex carbohydrates that were not absorbed earlier in the digestive process. Although humans do not have the enzymes to digest dietary fiber, bacteria do.

Fermentation is the breakdown of carbohydrates by bacteria. Energy is produced to keep the bacteria alive. Waste products of fermentation are short-chain fatty acids (SCFA), hydrogen gas, carbon dioxide gas, and, in some individuals, methane gas. Some of these gases are, in turn, consumed by other bacteria in the colon, yielding acetate, methane, sulfates, and hydrogen sulfide. Unused gasses are absorbed and excreted in the breath or excreted through the anus as flatulence. Most people produce one to four pints of gas a day and pass gas as flatulence up to 14 times per day.

It is important to remember that bacterial fermentation of dietary fiber is basically normal and desirable, at least to a point. The short-chain fatty acids produced by bacteria in your gut are important to your health and serve as the primary nutrients for the epithelial cells lining the colon. SCFAs may play important roles in the prevention of cancer and cardiovascular disease.

Some carbohydrates are fermented more rapidly than others, but FODMAPs are *all* rapidly fermentable. They make it possible for bacteria to produce a lot of gas in a short amount of time, causing abdominal pain, bloating, and excessive flatulence for some IBS sufferers. There is also some evidence that individuals with IBS may produce more gas from consuming FODMAPs than other people, and that people with different types of IBS produce different types of gas.

Some FODMAPs are specifically added to foods to stimulate fermentation by so-called good bacteria and to aid the production of short chain fatty acids. These additives are sometimes termed prebiotics, and include inulin and fructo-oligosaccharides (FOS). Unfortunately, they may increase symptoms due to rapid fermentation and increased gas production in some individuals. The term "prebiotic" is not to be confused with "probiotic." *Pro*biotics are the "good bacteria" that are sometime deliberately ingested for purported health benefits. *Pre*biotics are preferred carbohydrate foods for those good bacteria; many prebiotics are FODMAPs. Some supplements and foods contain both to stimulate increased activity of the good bacteria.

*Hydrogen Breath Testing*

A laboratory test called hydrogen breath testing is based on the fact that fermentation of malabsorbed carbohydrates results in bacterial production of excess hydrogen and/or methane gas. The gas is absorbed into the bloodstream and excreted in the breath, where it can be measured.

Your physician can order breath testing to check for fructose malabsorption. Fructose is only one of the FODMAPs, so why is it often singled out? Why is it helpful to know whether you malabsorb fructose? Screening for fructose malabsorption turns out to be one of the best ways to identify people who are likely to be helped by the FODMAP Elimination Diet. Not everyone with IBS malabsorbs fructose. Of those who do, however, studies suggest that up to 75% respond to a FODMAP-controlled diet with reduced symptoms. On the other hand, a negative test for fructose malabsorption may give the IBS sufferer more confidence consuming a varied diet, including fruit. Breath testing for lactose malabsorption is also available and can be ordered by your health care provider.

Studies have shown that not everyone who malabsorbs fructose or lactose experiences IBS symptoms. It is likely that other factors, such as visceral hypersensitivity, must also be present for symptoms to occur. For this reason, the results of these tests need to be considered in combination with the patient's history and symptoms of intolerance in order to diagnose or rule out fructose or lactose malabsorption.

In Australia and New Zealand, IBS patients are routinely screened for fructose malabsorption. At some medical centers there, patients who test positive for both IBS and fructose malabsorption are immediately referred for dietary counseling to reduce intake of fructose and other FODMAPs.

In the U.S., we are now beginning to see more testing for fructose malabsorption, but the practice is far from widespread. Even if you don't have access to a breath test, you can learn a lot about your ability to tolerate fructose and lactose by trying the FODMAP Elimination Diet program. Your response to the diet should tell you a great deal about whether you have a problem absorbing fructose.

Fructose malabsorption may be primary (occurring on its own, probably due to genetics) or secondary. Primary fructose malabsorption occurs in a person with a very slow rate of fructose absorption in an otherwise healthy intestinal tract and is usually genetic. Secondary fructose malabsorption could occur as a result of another disease process that damages or shortens the small intestine, or speeds up motility so that fructose is rushed through the small intestine before it has a chance to be absorbed.

## Understanding FODMAP Carbohydrates

As you learned earlier, FODMAP stands for Fermentable Oligo-, Di- and Mono-saccharides And Polyols. Specifically, the dietary carbohydrates described by the term FODMAP are lactose, fructose, fructans, polyols, and galactans/GOS. This section provides more details about each of these.

*Lactose*

Lactose is the primary sugar present in milk. It is a disaccharide of glucose and galactose. Lact*ose* is broken down by the enzyme lact*ase* in the small intestine before its component sugars are absorbed. Many people don't produce enough lactase and can't break down all the ingested lactose to glucose and galactose for full absorption. This lactase insufficiency can be primary or secondary.

Primary lactase insufficiency is very rare in infants and young children, who must be able to digest milk sugar in order to survive. However, up to 90% of adults produce significantly less lactase than in childhood, particularly those of African, Jewish, Native-American, Mexican, and Asian descent. In parts of the world (especially northern Europe) where the climate allows dairy cows to be raised, milk and milk products are a major part of the economy and cuisine. Interestingly, people descended from the northern European gene pool tend to retain the ability to digest lactose into adulthood, at least to some degree.

Secondary lactase insufficiency can result from any disease process that damages or removes the lactase-producing cells lining the small intestine, such as untreated celiac disease, gastroenteritis, Crohn's disease, or short bowel syndrome. It can also occur from any disease process that speeds up transit time to the point where lactose passes through the small intestine before it has time to be digested and absorbed, even if that disease does not directly affect the small intestine (ulcerative colitis, for example).

Ordinary milk contains 11-15 grams of lactose in a one-cup serving. Fermented milk products such as yogurt and kefir usually have less lactose because the bacteria in those products break down some of it, although they can have more, if whey and whey solids are added during processing. Untreated milk, yogurt, and kefir are not allowed on the Elimination Phase of the diet.

Hard cheeses have little or no lactose. During the cheese-making process, the whey is drained off the curds. Lactose is part of the whey, so most of it is removed from the cheese during this step. During aging, friendly microbes tend to consume any remaining lactose. Sour cream and butter have only a trace of lactose.

Lactose-free milk and milk products have been pre-treated with the enzyme lactase. The enzyme breaks lactose down to its simple sugars, and the resulting products are 100% lactose-free. Several brands are widely available in grocery stores in the U.S. and Canada. Even if the front of the label says the product is lactose-free, do check ingredients to make sure the product doesn't contain other FODMAPs.

Prescription drugs are an under-recognized source of lactose. Lactose is used as a filler or coating in approximately 20% of prescription drugs and 6% of over-the counter drugs. Ironically, this is true even for drugs meant to treat gastrointestinal diseases and disorders, including certain antispasmodics; anti-diarrheal tablets such as Imodium®; IBD drugs such as mesalazine, budesonide, and prednisolone; and pancreatin enzymes. People who take multiple medications might be consuming quite a bit of lactose in this way. While some people may be able to tolerate a gram or more of lactose each day in medications, others may not.

*Fructose*

Fructose is a simple sugar or monosaccharide. Intake of fructose in the U.S. has climbed significantly since 1970, when high-fructose corn syrup began to replace sucrose as the preferred sweetener in the food industry. Consumption rose from an estimated 8.8% of calories in the 1970s to 11.5% of calories by the 1990s.

Other factors in modern society, such as year-round access to high-quality fruit and easy access to sweeteners of all kinds, have also increased our fructose intake compared to the days before modern transportation, food processing, and storage methods. As recently as a hundred years ago, your ancestors probably had access to only local fruit in season along with what they could dry or can. Procuring honey meant finding a bees' nest, wresting the honeycomb from the bees, and extracting it, not driving to the grocery store to buy a jar.

"Free" fructose is found in honey, high-fructose corn syrup, and fruits. The ratio of fructose to glucose varies and is unique in each of these foods. Fructose can also be bound together with glucose in the form sucrose (table sugar), which contains an equal amount of fructose and glucose.

When the amount of fructose is equal to the amount of glucose in a food, it is absorbed more completely. That is why it is OK to eat small portions of certain fruits and table sugar on the FODMAP Elimination Phase. However, the rate at which fructose absorption occurs is slow and varies from one person to the next. Even though fructose and glucose are balanced in such foods, large portions can still overwhelm absorptive capacity and cause symptoms for sensitive individuals.

Therefore, on the allowed food lists for the Elimination Phase, you will find that the serving sizes for fruits and sweets of all kinds are limited.

During a FODMAP Elimination Diet, foods with *excess* fructose need to be avoided completely during the Elimination Phase. How do we define excess fructose? Foods with excess fructose have .2 grams more fructose than glucose per serving. In most cases that is less than a one percent difference.

Some in the food industry would have you believe that there is really no difference between high-fructose corn syrup and granulated sugar (which is always exactly 50% fructose). Yes, they are both sugars; yes, they both contain a combination of glucose and fructose; and yes, they can both contribute to obesity in excess—but there are some differences between them that are important to people with IBS.

According to the Corn Refiners Association, HFCS is sold to the food manufacturing industry principally in three formulations: 42% fructose, 55% fructose and 90% fructose. In fact, the 42% fructose version of HFCS does **not** have excess free fructose and would be permitted during the Elimination Phase of the FODMAP Elimination Diet. The 55% and 90% fructose versions clearly **do** meet the definition of excess free fructose and are capable of causing symptoms for some individuals.

Since ingredient listings on food labels don't identify which form of HFCS is in a given food or beverage, my advice is to avoid all forms of HFCS during the Elimination Phase of the diet. Feel free to include any and all HFCS during the fructose Challenge Phase of your diet. If the Corn Refiners Association is successful in its current bid to use the term "corn sugar" instead of the term "high-fructose corn syrup," the same will be true for foods with that ingredient. Note that ordinary light corn syrup does not contain excess fructose, and should be well tolerated by FODMAP-sensitive individuals.

It is likewise impossible to tell from reading the food label whether a high- or low-fructose version of "brown rice syrup" has been used, so that ingredient is not recommended.

*Fructans*

Fructans, a type of oligosaccharide, are chains of the sugar fructose. These chains vary in length, and it is the shorter and medium chains that are defined as FODMAPs because they are rapidly fermented and osmotically active. Short-chain fructans are often referred to as fructo-oligosaccharides (FOS). Inulins, which have slightly longer chains, are also FODMAPs. The fructan content of grains such as wheat varies with the variety of wheat, the growing conditions, and even the bread baking temperature and duration.

Because humans do not produce enzymes capable of breaking the fructose-fructose bonds present in fructans, they are not digested and absorbed in the small intestine.

The top food sources of fructans in the U.S. diet are wheat, onions, and garlic. Wheat alone supplies approximately 70% of those fructans, due to heavy consumption of bread, pizza, bagels, cereals, pasta, crackers, and baked goods by Americans. Rye is not prominent in the U.S. diet but is a significant source of FODMAPs in northern Europe.

Wheat is such a staple for most Americans that they never suspect it could be causing their symptoms; this culprit is hiding in plain sight. In fact, clients may say, "How could the problem be wheat? I eat wheat products every day, and some days I feel fine!" Many of these folks have managed their symptoms until now by eating a diet with limited amounts of fruits, vegetables, milk, and beans. While that may help symptoms drop back to a manageable level because it reduces the total FODMAP load, it leaves a diet with a limited range of nutrients and a lot of empty calories.

If you discover that wheat causes your IBS symptoms to worsen, you will have learned something very important. It probably will not mean that you can never have wheat again, but that you must choose the type, amount, and frequency of wheat intake very carefully and deliberately, to keep your IBS symptoms under control.

Inulin, sometimes also described on food labels as "chicory root extract," is sometimes added to foods and beverages, particularly certain yogurts, kefirs, breakfast cereals, and snack bars. The purpose of this food additive is to boost the fiber content of the food as a selling point and, in some cases, to promote the growth of "good" bacteria in the gut. FOS may be added to some products for the same reason. Obviously, this practice is unhelpful to many IBS sufferers.

### Polyols

Because the chemical structure of polyols resembles both sugars and alcohols, they are often called sugar alcohols. Polyols exhibit intense osmotic activity and are strong laxatives in large doses, even for people without IBS. This characteristic is often deliberately exploited and largely explains the reputation of prunes for preventing simple constipation.

Sorbitol, one type of polyol, occurs naturally in some fruits; in addition to prunes and apples, it is found in pears, blackberries, figs, dates, apricots, nectarines, peaches, plums, and cherries.

Many vegetables contain a naturally occurring polyol called mannitol. A few of the vegetables that contain the most mannitol are mushrooms, cauliflower, sweet corn, and snow peas.

Other polyols, derived from corn, sugar cane, or whey, are used as additives to sweeten sugarless gum, candy, and low-carb meal replacement bars. The list of ingredients in such foods might include xylitol, sorbitol, mannitol, maltitol, erythritol, isomalt, lactitol, or hydrogenated starch hydrolysates. Polydextrose, while not a sugar alcohol, is derived from sorbitol and has FODMAP properties. Erythritol may be an exception, as studies show it is well absorbed by humans.

The presence of polyols in the food or meal worsens fructose absorption. Individuals who malabsorb fructose may have an especially difficult time tolerating apples and pears, which are high in both free fructose and sorbitol.

Some liquid medications are sweetened with polyols. If you take liquid medications on a regular basis, check with your pharmacist to find out what your medication is sweetened with, and whether the medication is available in another form. Never discontinue a prescribed liquid medication without the guidance of the prescribing physician.

### Galactans/GOS

Galactans are also known as galacto-oligosaccharides (GOS). Galactans, like fructans, are a type of oligosaccharide. Galactans are chains of the sugar galactose. The primary dietary sources of galactans are legumes (pulses), such as baked beans, kidney beans, chickpeas, soy beans, and lentils. While legumes (pulses) are a valuable source of nutrients for all of us, if we can tolerate them, they are of much more significance in the diet of vegetarians.

Galactans, like fructans, are not absorbed in the small intestine because humans do not produce an enzyme capable of breaking the galactose-galactose bond. Galactans in the large intestine are highly fermentable and osmotically active. They can be relied on to cause gas, and they give beans their reputation as the "musical fruit." Most people with FODMAP intolerance will be working to simply establish tolerable portions sizes of galactan-containing foods.

# Chapter 5: Frequently Asked Questions (FAQ)

*Q. What do you mean by food chemicals?*

Some food chemicals occur naturally in food or beverages, such as caffeine, amines, salicylates, or solanine. Others are added to processed foods, such as food dyes, MSG, benzoic, or citric acid. It is outside the scope of this book to address food chemical sensitivities.

*Q. How can I learn more about food sensitivities that involve my immune system?*

An allergist, usually a medical doctor or osteopath, can test you for what I would call "classic food allergies," for example, allergy to peanuts or eggs. These allergies can be triggered by small amounts of ingested food and have immediate and potentially severe adverse effects, including hives, swelling of the mouth and throat, and anaphylactic shock.

There are other types of adverse food reaction, also involving your immune system, that are often delayed, and are more "dosage sensitive" than classic food allergies; the more of the food or food chemical you consume, the stronger the reaction. Examples of food chemicals are caffeine, amines, sulfites, nitrates, salicylates, artificial colors, and preservatives. It is possible, although outside the scope of this book, to find lists of foods containing these chemicals, so that you can avoid them. However, in my practice I find it is more effective to recommend special blood tests, such as the Mediator Release Test by Signet Diagnostic Corporation; the test results are a valuable tool for planning the patient's diet and reducing symptoms due to food chemical sensitivies. See www.ibsfree.net for more information about Mediator Release Testing (MRT®) and the LEAP® diet.

*Q. How can I find a dietitian to help me with the FODMAP Elimination Diet program?*

If your doctor can't provide a referral, please see the "FODMAP-Friendly Dietitian" link on my blog, www.ibsfree.net. These dietitians have volunteered their contact information and their interest in working with IBS/FODMAP clients. Although I have not verified their credentials or experience, a growing number of registered dietitians are prepared to help you. You will get better counseling from your dietitian if you express your interest in a

FODMAP Elimination Diet at the time you make your appointment. If you need additional help locating a dietitian in your area, you can use the Academy of Nutrition and Dietetics' Find a Dietitian tool at www.eatright.org.

*Q. My doctor says diet doesn't matter with IBS and I can eat anything I want. Why would she say such a thing?*

Patients often report hearing variations of this as they wake up, groggy, from their colonoscopies. At this moment, the doctor is feeling pleased that he or she does not have to report any dire findings to you. In her mind is, "thank goodness it's only IBS" and not cancer or Crohn's disease. Your doctor knows that IBS is not a lethal disease. If she has never been in your shoes, she may not appreciate how IBS symptoms can sometimes seem to control your life. Knowing that a varied diet is important, your doctor may not want to see you limit your diet unnecessarily. If you are underweight, she may just want you to eat, period. I like to think of it as a well meaning but imprecise way to say, "There is no one-size-fits-all diet for IBS."

As a nutritionist, of course, I strongly believe that what we eat does matter! It seems obvious that the gastrointestinal tract would be affected physically by food as it is digested and absorbed. Nutrients are not merely building blocks for body tissues; they also act as chemical messengers to every cell in our bodies. In addition to feeding us, they feed our commensal gut bacteria.

If I could put words in the doctor's mouth, I would suggest something like this: "It's important to eat the most varied diet possible. However, some people with IBS find that certain foods set off their symptoms. Your project will be to work out which foods will nourish your body, yet keep your symptoms to a minimum." While I am entertaining this little scenario, let me go one step further. Next, the doctor will say, "I'd like to refer you to a registered dietitian to help you sort this out." You don't have to wait for the doctor to suggest a referral. You can ask your primary care or gastrointestinal doctor to recommend a dietitian. Or, you can just contact a registered dietitian directly and make an appointment.

*Q. What does the medical literature say about fiber therapy for IBS?*

Eight recent reviews uniformly concluded that fiber therapy has little or no benefit for most IBS patients. Results of a clinical trial published in the British Journal of Medicine in 2009 found that for one patient to attain adequate relief of abdominal pain or discomfort during the first month of treatment, between four (psyllium) and 33 (bran) patients must be treated with fiber supplements! Television, Internet, and print advertising to the contrary, only one out of 11 patients treated with all kinds of fiber supplements experiences prevention of persistent symptoms.

*Q. Why does my doctor insist on calling my fructose malabsorption (FM) "fructose intolerance"—doesn't he know any better?*

Patients with dietary fructose intolerance seem to strongly prefer the term FM to describe their condition, to avoid confusing it with hereditary fructose intolerance. However, the term "dietary fructose intolerance" or even "fructose intolerance" continues to be an accurate medical description of the symptoms that result from fructose malabsorption, in the same way that lactose intolerance results from lactose malabsorption. Health care provider using those terms are neither ignorant nor uncaring about the needs of the patient with FM.

*Q. Why do FODMAPs cause IBS symptoms for some people and not for others?*

There are a number of factors that may explain why FODMAPs cause more troublesome symptoms for some people than for others. For example, individuals vary a great deal in how much lactase they produce, with more than half of adults having reduced lactase activity. Lactase is the enzyme needed to break milk sugar down into two smaller sugars for absorption. Without it, undigested milk sugar is presented to the bacteria in the large intestine, where it acts as a source of food for them. Some, but not all, lactase-deficient people can usually tolerate a few grams of lactose in one sitting. In combination with the other FODMAPs, however, even smaller amounts may cause difficulty.

Unlike lactose, fructose and sugar alcohols aren't malabsorbed because of enzyme deficiency; fructose and sugar alcohol absorption are just naturally slow processes. Some of us absorb the large loads of fructose and sugar alcohols in today's modern diet less efficiently than others, so our malabsorption is normal to some extent. Unabsorbed fructose and polyols that are delivered to the large intestine can cause chaos when they are digested by the resident bacteria. Likewise, it is normal for fructans (found in certain grains, fruits, and vegetables) and galactans/GOS (found in beans and some vegetables) to be undigested and unabsorbed in the small intestine. Being essentially indigestible is part of what defines them as fiber.

People with more adaptable bowels are not bothered by symptoms when consuming these foods unless they eat an unusually large portion, and may in fact use these foods deliberately to "stay regular." Those with less adaptable bowels may experience IBS symptoms after consuming these foods. In some individuals, the nervous system serving the gut is more sensitive and responds with pain to gut distention.

On another note, some individuals have such a fast intestinal transit time that FODMAPs do not have a chance to be absorbed before being presented to the bacteria in the large intestine. Others have slow intestinal transit time. There is some evidence that constipation is associated with the presence of methane in the breath of affected individuals. Breath methane would likely be the result of methane-producing bacteria in the large intestine. It is not clear yet what this means, but it may somehow influence why some people with IBS have constipation and others do not.

Finally, some people may have small intestinal bacterial overgrowth (SIBO). Bacteria growing inappropriately in the small intestine may have access to fermentable carbohydrates before they have had a chance to be absorbed.

Some or all of the above factors may cause IBS symptoms in a single person. The FODMAP Elimination Diet has the potential to improve symptoms caused by all of them, by depriving the gut bacteria of their favorite foods.

*Q. What is the difference between a FODMAP Elimination Diet and a FODMAP-restricted diet?*

Though it might seem like splitting hairs, there is actually an important difference between these two concepts. The phrase "elimination diet" has a very specific meaning—it is a strict, temporary, regimen that we follow to learn what foods or food categories trigger symptoms. You will learn how to do a FODMAP Elimination Diet in this book.

A FODMAP-restricted diet is what you will do after you learn what your problem areas are, with the ultimate goal of enjoying the most liberal, varied diet possible. It is simply a low-FODMAP diet. If you don't have the inclination to do the whole elimination diet program, you could use the alternate approach described in Chapter 3 to a do a FODMAP-restricted diet from the outset.

*Q. My doctor wants me to take a fiber supplement. Which one should I take and when should I take it?*

This is a question to discuss directly with your health care provider. Although statistics show that most people don't benefit from fiber therapy, there is a small chance you will be the one who does. If the health care provider who knows you best wants you to take a fiber supplement, you should give it a fair trial.

Theoretically, non-fermentable fibers such as those based on cellulose would be FODMAP-friendly, though to my knowledge these products have not been analyzed for FODMAPs. If you already use another fiber supplement and you aren't happy with the results, you may want to consider switching to Citrucel® or Fiber-Con® before starting the Elimination Phase of the FODMAP Elimination Diet. Their manufacturers claim that these are 100% non-fermentable—in other words, not FODMAPs. If your system is very sensitive, you can accomplish this by using a little less of your current fiber supplement each day over a week's time until you are down to nothing. At the same time, starting with the lowest dose of the new fiber supplement (check the product label for details), gradually increase over a week's time until you are using an effective dose of the product. If you choose to change fiber supplements, do it before starting the diet. Try not to start a new fiber supplement in the middle of the elimination diet process.

Studies show that psyllium husk supplements (Konsyl® or Metamucil Fiber Powder®) may be helpful for treatment of chronic constipation, though they are fermentable and may cause increased bloating and gas in some individuals. Wheat dextrin (Benefiber®) has a fermentation profile similar to inulin (Metamucil Clear and Natural®). Again, these products have not been specifically analyzed for FODMAPs, to my knowledge.

Acacia fiber (the source of gum arabic), ground flax (linseeds), chia, and hemp seeds are popular sources of fiber in today's Internet marketplace, but none has been well-studied for effectiveness in the treatment of IBS. They have not been analyzed specifically for complete FODMAP composition as of this writing. Rice bran and oat bran are relatively low in FODMAPs and can contribute fiber to the diet.

To summarize, it is best to get your fiber from intact low-FODMAP foods. However, if you must take a fiber supplement, and the first one you try doesn't help, try one of another type. If you use seeds, be sure they are ground. When starting a new fiber supplement, start with a small dose and work up to the full labeled dose over time. If the prescribed fiber supplement doesn't help, or if it makes you feel worse, discuss discontinuing it with your health care provider.

*Q. Can vegetarians use this diet?*

Yes. At first glance, it may seem difficult for vegetarians to get enough protein during the Elimination Phase of the FODMAP diet, but it can be done with careful attention to detail. Lacto-ovo vegetarians will have an easier time of it than vegans, and should have no difficulty getting by for a couple of weeks during the trial using lactose-free milk products, eggs, nuts, seeds, green peas, tofu and quinoa as protein sources. It is important to monitor your diet to ensure that you are consuming at least 46 grams of protein each day for women and at least 56 grams of protein each day for men. These are guidelines for young and middle aged adults in good health. If you are elderly or have any other medical conditions please consult your health care provider about how much protein is safe and appropriate for you.

Non-celiac vegetarians can use a meat substitute known as seitan in place of soy products. It is easy to make from vital wheat gluten and contains about 26 grams of protein per half cup serving. See here for some more vegetarian meal ideas.

*Q. I have fructose malabsorption (FM). Does the material in this book apply to me?*

Certainly the sections that directly relate to fructose apply to you. It is common for individuals with fructose malabsorption or dietary fructose intolerance to have other carbohydrate intolerances as well. The FODMAP Elimination Diet is a way to explore whether you can also benefit from reducing other highly fermentable, osmotically active carbohydrates in your diet.

*Q. How does this program compare to the Atkins Diet?*

The Atkins Diet is a very low-carbohydrate diet. The FODMAP Elimination Diet is not. Rather, it is a carbohydrate-controlled diet, with the major focus on the type of carbohydrate. There is no limit on total carbohydrate intake as there is with the Atkins Diet.

*Q. How does this program compare to the Specific Carbohydrate Diet (SCD) and the Gut and Psychology Syndrome Diet (GAPS)?*

These three diet programs, FODMAPs, SCD, and GAPS, share a common thread. They are all based on the belief that each person's health and well being is heavily impacted by his or her gut microflora. They attempt to influence the activity of the gut bacteria by controlling the types of food, particularly carbohydrates, in the diet. The SCD and GAPs diets were not designed specifically to treat IBS symptoms; they aim to have a more global effect on the physical and mental health of the individual as the result of changes in diet.

There are a number of specific variations in the foods that are allowed on the three protocols. But more importantly, there is a philosophical difference regarding adherence to the diets. Compared to the FODMAP Elimination Diet, SCD and GAPS require long-term commitment and fundamental changes in food sourcing, purchasing, meal planning, and preparation. The authors of the SCD and GAPS diets suggest that only absolute adherence to the diet over an extended period of time can restore the individual to health. Experimentation or variations from the dietary principles are strongly discouraged.

The FODMAP elimination protocol described in this book takes a more experimental approach. Food challenges and dietary experimentation begin after the initial Elimination Phase of just a few weeks. "Problem foods" can be consumed in moderation, instead of being considered "illegal." The aim of the FODMAP Elimination Diet is to limit IBS symptoms to a tolerable level, as determined by the client. Perhaps this is not as ambitious as the cures to which Dr. Gottschall (SCD) and Dr. Natasha Campbell-McBride (GAPS) aspire. It seems there may be a place for all of these approaches, depending on the medical condition, resources, and values of the individual.

*Q. How does this program compare to the Paleo diet?*

The logic behind the Paleolithic diet is that humans aren't meant to eat foods that would not have been available to our caveman ancestors, such as grains, legumes (pulses), out-of season fruits, processed sugars, and oils. Many FODMAPs are automatically eliminated by most variations of the Paleo diet, so it probably works pretty well to manage IBS for a lot of people. I especially appreciate that limited access to sweeteners throughout most of human history should probably guide current practice. But I think that humans are essentially opportunistic feeders and are meant to eat any food they can tolerate, so it doesn't make sense to me that one should not eat rice or potatoes or milk or any other category of food without consideration of individual tolerance.

*Q. How does this program compare to treatment approaches that rely heavily on soluble fiber from food and acacia fiber supplements?*

High-fiber programs may help a small minority of individuals with IBS. However, such high-fiber diets for everyone with IBS are not consistent with current medical literature. Eight recent reviews uniformly concluded that fiber either has no efficacy for treatment of IBS or has possible limited benefits for patients who have IBS with constipation. Today we know that across-the-board "high-fiber, "low-fat" and "no red meat" diets for IBS are not necessary for everyone with IBS.

*Q. Does fructose or lactose malabsorption cause depression?*

Several very small studies have shown a link between carbohydrate malabsorption, lower levels of tryptophan, zinc, and folate in the blood, and depressive symptoms, particularly in females. But the studies simply weren't designed to prove that fructose and/or lactose malabsorption cause depression. There are far more questions than answers here, yet it does not appear to be an active area of research at this time. That hasn't stopped the idea from taking on a life of its own, and it is treated as fact on a number of web sites and blogs.

What is the take-away message here for people with fructose and/or lactose malabsorption? If you're a woman, there is a chance that removing excess amounts of these sugars from your diet might make you feel better mentally as well as physically.

*Q. Will FODMAP elimination help my gastroesophageal reflux disease (GERD)?*

Theoretically, it might offer some relief. The large bowel (colon) wraps all the way around the abdominal cavity and passes close by the stomach in the upper abdomen. If the colon is distended with fluid and gas due to FODMAPs ingestion, it could put some physical pressure on the stomach. The upward pressure might encourage reflux of the stomach contents into the esophagus, as it does during pregnancy. We might guess this effect would be more likely in people with a lot of abdominal body fat or short-waisted body types.

*Q. I don't like/can't get some of the foods on your sample menus. What else can I have?*

You can substitute any of the other foods that are allowed on the Elimination Phase of the diet. Here are a few ideas, which you can scale up to meet your appetite and calorie needs. The serving sizes of the bold items must stay small, however:

### Breakfast Ideas:

1 egg, scrambled with lactose-free milk
½ C. grits
1 t. butter
**1 clementine**

1 C. cream of rice, buckwheat, quinoa flakes, hot cereal/porridge
½ C. lactose-free milk
**2 T. toasted almond slivers**

Gluten-free pancake or waffle
2 t. butter
**1 ½ T. 100% pure maple syrup**

1 C. cornflakes, crispy rice/rice bubbles, rice or corn Chex, puffed
   rice, millet, quinoa or amaranth, Cheerios (check labels for all of
   these—ingredients may vary by region)
1 C. lactose-free milk, rice milk or almond milk
**½ C. sliced strawberries**

Smoothie with 1 C. lactose-free yogurt or kefir, **½ C. frozen
   strawberries**, ½ C. ice cubes and 1 scoop rice protein powder
   (check ingredients)

### Lunch or Dinner Ideas

2 C. homemade chicken and rice soup, including ½ C. allowed
   vegetables
4 rice crackers
**1 kiwi**

2 C. homemade vegetable beef soup, including ½ C. allowed
   vegetables
3 rice cakes
**½ C. grapes**

2 C. homemade fish chowder, including 1 C. lactose-free milk, ½
   C. potatoes and ½ C. allowed vegetables

Quesadillas, including 2 corn tortilla with 2 oz. low-fat cheddar
   cheese

½ C. carrots sticks
1 C. lactose-free milk

3 oz. baked cod with olive oil and herbs
½ C. polenta
½ C. steamed spinach with butter and vinegar

3 oz. grilled salmon with wedge of lemon
½ C. each grilled cherry tomatoes and zucchini
1 C. rice

3 oz. lean beef steak or hamburger
½ C. mashed potatoes made with butter and lactose-free milk
½ C. sautéed red bell pepper

3 oz. lobster with butter
1½ C. corn pasta salad, including ½ C. allowed vegetables and
    mayonnaise

1½ C. macaroni and cheese, made with corn/quinoa pasta, lactose-
    free milk, and cheddar cheese
½ C. caramelized carrots

3 oz. turkey
½ C. mashed potatoes made with butter and lactose-free milk
½ C. acorn squash
**¼ C. homemade cranberry and orange relish**

3 oz. grilled steak
2 corn tortillas, skillet warmed
½ C. sautéed red pepper strips
½ C. chopped tomato
**1½ T. sour cream**

3 oz. peeled shrimp
1 C. vegetable soup, including ½ C. allowed vegetables
14 rice crackers

*Q. Do you have some meal ideas for vegetarians?*

Try some of these ideas in place of the meat items on the sample menus:

- Millet-potato bread with nut butter and sliced banana
- Zucchini frittata
- Brown rice tortilla warmed with shredded cheese, stuffed with lettuce, tomato, feta cheese, and olives, drizzled with tahini and lemon juice
- Cooked rice, stir-fried with carrots, celery, red peppers, and seitan or tofu (recipe)

*Q. I eat out a lot. What can I order at restaurants that will work on this diet?*

Although you will find it easier to prepare your food at home, dining out can still be done on the FODMAP Elimination Diet. Grilled salmon, steak, and chicken are widely available, and the ubiquitous sides of baked potato or rice are FODMAP-friendly. Order a side salad with oil and vinegar (hold the onions), and you are all set. If you prefer more adventurous fare, you are in luck. Many world cuisines are rice based, such as Thai, Chinese, Japanese, and Indian. Have a look at the menu and choose some sort of grilled or roasted beef, chicken, shrimp, or fish with traditional seasonings. Add rice or rice noodles with an assortment of steamed or stir-fried vegetables, hold the onions. The sauces are likely to contain most of the FODMAPs in these meals; ask for them on the side so you can use just a little or none at all. Here are some additional ideas

**Airport, highway, or convenience store:** Starbucks or McDonald's oatmeal, Wendy's baked potato, sushi, banana, small fresh fruit cup, handful of roasted nuts, Italian ice or sorbet (check sweetener), tortilla chips, sliced deli meat, chicken or tuna salad, prepared grilled chicken salad, chef salad or chicken Caesar salad (skip the croutons), hard boiled eggs, cheese, pumpkin seeds/pepitas, macadamia nuts, peanuts, pickles

**Breakfast:** Oatmeal/porridge (prepared with water), banana or small fresh fruit cup (usually mostly melon, grapes and strawberries), eggs (any style), bacon or sausage, hash brown potatoes, grits

**American:** Broth-based soup; grilled steak, fish, or chicken (not breaded or fried); salad with oil and vinegar (hold the onions); baked potato with butter and sour cream; plain rice; steamed or sautéed beets, carrots, spinach, squash

**Asian:** Egg drop soup; chicken satay with peanut sauce; white or brown rice; rice noodles; sweet and sour chicken or tofu and vegetables (if sauce is restaurant-prepared with sugar); fresh spring rolls (rice paper wrapper), sushi (if such rice is seasoned with sugar); grilled fish, chicken, or beef teriyaki

**Italian**: Antipasto plate; salad with oil and vinegar; chicken or fish on a bed of steamed spinach; Italian ice

**Indian:** Tandoori chicken, rice

**Mediterranean:** Chicken, beef, or lamb kebabs; grilled red pepper, zucchini, tomatoes; rice

**Mexican:** Tortilla chips; quesadilla on corn tortilla; chicken, fish, beef, or pork enchilada, taco, or fajita with corn tortilla; grilled red peppers, plain rice

*Q. My health care provider wants me to gain weight—which foods on the FODMAP Elimination Phase would be useful for this purpose?*

Underweight or malnourished IBS sufferers should seek assistance from a registered dietitian to plan for weight gain. The following ideas are provided for educational purposes only:

It is helpful to recall that oils do not contain any FODMAP carbohydrates, and that oils are high in calories compared to other foods. So the number one weight gain strategy for FODMAP sensitive individuals is to eat more healthy fats, such as olive oil, any kind of nut or seed oil, and peanut or almond butter. I know, I know, you've always read that people with IBS shouldn't eat too much fat, but is that really true for you? Try it and see for yourself, before you limit your fat intake unnecessarily, based on over-generalized advice. Maybe it's true, maybe it's not; you might be able to tolerate more fat than you think. There is a huge difference between a tablespoon of olive oil (13.5 grams of fat) and a Bloomin' Onion® (134 grams of fat). Just because fried foods make you feel sick, might not mean you can't put olive oil on your salad or drizzle your roasted veggies liberally with oil. Also, some people mistakenly think it is the fat in the food that bothers them when it is really the bread, pasta, or vegetable the fat was applied to that was the problem.

Foods high in protein are the next best low-FODMAP source of calories for weight gain, again because they are automatically low in both sugars and fibers. If you need to gain weight, and you don't have any other health issues such as kidney stones or kidney disease that would make it inadvisable to eat more protein, your dietitian might suggest eating more of the following foods from the Allowed Meats/Milk section of the elimination diet:

Beef
Pork
Chicken
Fish
Seafood
Tofu
Lactose-free milk
Lactose-free yogurt or kefir or smoothies
Lactose-free cottage cheese
Hard Cheeses
Eggs
Puddings and custards made with lactose-free milk, eggs, and granulated sugar
Macaroni and cheese made with corn pasta, cheddar cheese, and lactose-free milk

You must try these things for yourself to see if you tolerate them. Don't over-restrict based on one-size-fits-all advice you may have read or heard about what people with IBS should or shouldn't eat.

*Q. I need to lose some weight. Can I use the FODMAP Elimination Diet for that?*

Even though the FODMAP Elimination Diet is not meant to be a weight loss plan, some people find they do experience some moderate weight loss on the Elimination Phase. Why? Because following the diet means they are eating less junk food and drinking fewer sweet beverages. If weight loss is one of your health care goals, here are a few tips:

- Most people who are trying to lose weight should limit "allowed extras" to about 100 calories per day.
- The sample menus in the book might provide more calories than you need, especially if you are sedentary, female, older, or of small stature. Try cutting back one serving from each food group. Don't consume less than 1200 calories without professional guidance—it is hard to get adequate nutrients on less than 1200 calories.
- Don't replace wheat-based baked goods with commercial gluten-free products, which tend to be loaded with calories, sugar, and fat. It is easier, cheaper, tastier, and healthier to just steer away from breads and baked goodies for a couple of weeks than to try replacing them.

- As usual, watch portions. Big bowls of white rice or wheat-free cookies might be FODMAP-friendly but can still provide too many calories for your needs.

- Exercise is a lot more fun when you don't have to worry about being within a 20-yard dash of the toilet! As your symptoms improve, maybe you will decide it's time to start an outdoor exercise program. Walking, biking, kayaking, hiking...they all can be yours again!

*Q. Why is there so much conflicting information about FODMAPs on the Internet?*

Please note that the food lists included in this edition of the book are, to the best of my knowledge, up-to-date at the time of printing. Without a doubt, the lists that are published today will need to be updated in the future.

There are a only a few labs producing full and original data on the FODMAP composition of food, most notably researchers at the Department of Medicine, Monash University, Box Hill Hospital, Australia. Do your best to determine whether the information you are evaluating is from a reputable source, based on the latest data, and using the most modern analytical methods.

Another reason for conflicting reports is that the FODMAP content of food is affected by its botanical variety, growing conditions, ripeness, storage, processing, preparation methods, and more. Just for starters, consider the natural difference in sweetness between an over-ripe and an under-ripe banana, or between a Granny Smith and a McIntosh apple. Think of all the different varieties of grapes grown for wine-making or the many varieties of apples for sale in your local grocery store, each one unique. Likewise, there are many varieties of corn, some grown for their sweetness (high in mannitol), and some grown for grinding into cornmeal or for popping. Consider the many different sweeteners that dried cranberries might be treated with. These are just a few of hundreds of examples.

As you evaluate the source of the information or advice you are reading, recognize that online support groups are peopled by generous individuals who reach out to help others based on their own experiences. Since sensitivity to FODMAPs varies so greatly from one person to the next, you need to remember that you are the final authority for how you feel before, during, and after your FODMAP Elimination Diet program. Don't limit your diet based on the opinion or experience of someone else without trying things out for yourself.

Conflicts can also seem to occur when either the writer or the reader is fuzzy on the context. It is one thing to be strictly following an elimination/challenge protocol, and it is another thing just to eat a "low-FODMAP" or FODMAP-restricted diet. A good example here might be Greek yogurt. No, it is not allowed on the Elimination Phase of this diet. Yes, you may read elsewhere that it is a good choice for a low-FODMAP diet because it is lower in lactose than other yogurts. All true. Remind yourself of your "elimination vs. low-FODMAP" status as you review confusing or seemingly contradictory information and be as clear as possible about your current goals.

My overall advice? Do not let small discrepancies, as irritating as they may be, distract you from the big picture. Just do your best to keep tabs on new information as it becomes available. Visit my blog at http://www.ibsfree.net to keep up with the latest on FODMAPs. Follow @CatsosIBSFreeRD on Twitter and "like" me on Facebook.

*Q. I'm going on vacation next week; should I start the diet now or wait till my holiday is over?*

If you have a few days before the holiday it might be worth the effort to get started right away. Wouldn't it be nice to have a vacation that isn't punctuated by anxiety about where to find the next toilet? If you will be off work at home or visiting your mom who wants to help you try some new recipes, it could be an ideal time to focus on your own health and nutrition. However, if you will be traveling and eating in restaurants or in other people's homes where you can't control the food, you might want to wait until after your schedule gets back to normal.

*Q. How soon can I eat another **bold** food?*

Give yourself two or three hours before eating another one.

*Q. Do I really have to stay on the Elimination Phase for two weeks if I feel better right away?*

Yes. IBS symptoms can vary from day to day, as you know. Two weeks will give you enough time to draw a more accurate conclusion about whether the diet has helped, particularly if constipation is part of your IBS picture.

*Q. Don't I need to know the exact number of grams of FODMAPs in all these foods?*

Most people with FODMAP intolerance are not sick because green bell peppers have .37 grams per 100 grams more sorbitol than red bell peppers. They are sick because their bodies can't handle large serving of milk, yogurt, ice cream, fruit, onions, garlic, or beans, and the modern diet contains too much bread, bagels, pasta, high-fiber bars and cereals, artificial sweeteners, sugary beverages, and juices.

Start by keeping your eyes on the big picture. Just enjoy eating the foods on these allowed food lists and take a break from scouring the Internet for minutiae. There is always time for that later if you turn out to be one of the unfortunate, FODMAP super-sensitive folks.

*Q. What about kale, or kumquats, or any one of the many foods that don't appear on the lists in this book?*

To be on the safe side, temporarily leave out these foods of unknown FODMAP content. If you'd like to try them later on, use the search function on www.ibsfree.net to review previous discussion about the food, or do some basic research to help you make an educated guess. For example, one can easily find reputable information placing kale in the cabbage family, so it is probably not allowed. Parsnips are root vegetables similar to carrots, so they are probably OK. Of course, these educated guesses will have to be revised to suit the facts when they become available.

*Q. I see one of my problem foods on the allowed lists. I could never eat that! What does this mean about the diet?*

Make sure your problem food isn't a "red herring." Are you absolutely certain you aren't confusing your problem food with other foods and beverages you usually eat at the same time? For example, a patient may notice that peanut butter is associated with symptoms later in the day. Upon further reflection, he realizes that he always eats peanut butter on bread or fresh apple slices, both high-FODMAP foods. The elimination diet protocol will help sort this situation out. However, if you are certain that you are allergic or otherwise unable to eat a food that appears on the "allowed" lists, simply cross that food off the list and do not eat it. There are many kinds of adverse reactions to food, and intolerance to FODMAP carbohydrates is just one of them.

*Q. Those portions are too small/too big for me. Can I eat more/less?*

You can eat portions dictated by your appetite and calorie needs except for foods shown in **bold type**. Do not eat larger portions of those foods during the Elimination Phase of the diet.

*Q. Do I have to worry about FODMAPs in my skin care or personal hygiene products?*

The answer is no, for skin care products. FODMAPs applied to your skin cannot get into your gut to produce symptoms by way of fermentation and disrupted fluid balance. While it is true that some food chemicals can be absorbed through the skin and potentially cause immune-mediated symptoms (e.g. salicylates), that is another story.

The answer is a little less clear for toothpaste and mouthwash. FODMAPs in these products can potentially be ingested. If you are not in the habit of swallowing your toothpaste, it's unlikely to cause a problem. However, if you learn you are particularly sensitive to sugar alcohols in your diet, you could consider seeking oral care products that do not contain them, to see if it makes a difference for you, as it has for some of my readers.

*Q. What can I use to replace fluids lost in diarrhea or excessive perspiration?*

Well, for heaven's sake, don't use regular milk, high-fructose corn syrup-sweetened soft drinks, or full strength fruit juice, as many of my patients have done. These remedies may be making matters worse because of their FODMAP content. If you are truly dehydrated, please contact your health care provider for medical advice. If you are simply looking for some everyday fluids that won't contribute to osmotic diarrhea, try some of the following: Quench® (by Clif); O-Water®; regular or herbal tea or iced tea with lemon and sugar; lime- or lemonade lightly sweetened with sugar; orange, grapefruit, or grape juice spritzer (a splash of juice in a cup of seltzer water); cucumber or lemon-infused water; lactose-free milk; homemade chicken or beef broth.

*Q. From years of trouble with my bowels, I am practically obsessed with getting enough fiber! How can I get enough fiber on this diet?*

Remember, if a high-fiber diet with fiber supplements were the cure for your IBS, you wouldn't be reading this book. I have seen patients who were eating as much as 70 grams of fiber per day in fruitless attempts to solve their IBS problems. Even at less extreme intakes, the high-fiber diet you've been told to consume in the past may be causing your symptoms, not helping to cure them. I recognize the benefits of dietary fiber as much as anyone, but the fact is not everyone can tolerate 30 or more grams of fiber. Give the elimination diet a chance to work, even if it seems different from what you are used to—that's the point!

Healthy women should aim for 21-26 grams of fiber per day, if tolerated; healthy men should aim for 30-38 grams of fiber per day, if tolerated.

On the other hand, if you are starting from a very low-fiber diet, you can add fiber in the form of whole grains, nuts, seeds, and allowed fruits and vegetables by very slowly increasing portions to give your body time to adjust.

Good sources of fiber on the FODMAP Elimination Diet include:

brown rice
rice bran
corn pasta and tortillas
oatmeal/porridge
oat bran
potatoes with skins
allowed fruits
allowed vegetables
nuts and nut butters
seeds and seed butters

*Q. Which foods are the best sources of vitamins and minerals?*

The best way to assure adequate intake of nutrients is to select a wide variety of foods from the Elimination Phase allowed foods. The following foods are particularly good sources of nutrients. One caveat here: vegetarians and vegans have their work cut out for them, because animal products are the best low-FODMAP sources of many vitamins and minerals. Because animal products are the only source in the case of vitamin B-12, vegans should take vitamin B-12 supplements.

**Food sources of vitamin A:**
Beet greens
Cantaloupe
Carrots and carrot juice
Collard greens
Fresh tomatoes
Green peas
Herring
Lettuce
Salmon
Spinach
Winter squash

**Food sources of vitamin C:**
Cantaloupe
Collard greens
Cranberries
Fresh tomatoes
Grapefruits and grapefruit juice
Kiwi
Lemons and lemon juice
Oranges and orange juice
Pineapple
Red bell peppers
Strawberries

**Food sources of vitamin D:**
Cod liver oil
Eggs
Flounder
Halibut
Herring
Pork
Rainbow trout
Salmon
Sole
Swordfish
Tuna
Vitamin D-fortified milk

**Food sources of vitamin E:**
Collard greens
Nuts, especially almonds
Quinoa
Spinach
Sunflower seeds
Sunflower, safflower and canola
    oil
Wild rice

**Food sources of vitamin K:**
Beet greens
Collard greens
Lettuce
Okra
Spinach
Turnip greens

**Food sources of folate:**
Beets
Collard greens

Spinach
Green peas
Lettuce
Mung bean sprouts
Okra
Oranges and orange juice
Quinoa
Sunflower seeds
Turnip greens

**Food sources of thiamine
    (vitamin B1):**
Carrots
Grapefruit
Green peas
Okra
Oranges
Pork
Potatoes with skin
Quinoa
Salmon

**Food sources of riboflavin
    (vitamin B2):**
Almonds
Beef
Eggs
Lactose-free cottage cheese
Lactose-free kefir
Lactose-free milk
Lactose-free yogurt
Pork
Quinoa
Spinach

**Food sources of niacin
    (vitamin B3):**
Haddock
Halibut
Ham
Pork
Potatoes with skin
Salmon
Tuna

**Food sources of vitamin B12:**
Beef
Clams
Crab
Eggs
Fish of all kinds
Lactose-free cottage cheese
Lactose-free kefir
Lactose-free milk
Lactose-free yogurt
Oysters
Pork
Poultry of all kinds

**Food sources of calcium:**
Canned salmon
Cheese
Collards
Lactose-free cottage cheese
Lactose-free kefir
Lactose-free milk
Lactose-free yogurt
Okra
Sardines
Spinach
Tofu
Turnip greens

**Food sources of iron:**
Baked potato with skin
Beef
Beets
Buckwheat
Cornmeal
Clams
Fish of all kinds
Mussels
Oysters
Pork and ham
Quinoa
Spinach

**Food sources of zinc:**
Beef
Chicken
Crab
Duck
Lamb
Oysters
Pork
Turkey

**Food sources of magnesium:**
Beef
Beet greens
Buckwheat
Cornmeal
Lactose-free cottage cheese
Lactose-free kefir
Lactose-free milk
Lactose-free yogurt
Nuts
Pork
Poultry
Pumpkin seeds/pepitas
Spinach

**Food sources of phosphorus:**
Crab
Eggs
Fish of all kinds
Lactose-free cottage cheese
Lactose-free kefir
Lactose-free milk
Lactose-free yogurt
Meat
Potatoes with skin
Poultry
Pumpkin seeds/pepitas
Quinoa
Sunflower seeds

**Food sources of potassium:**
Bananas
Cantaloupe
Carrots
Collard greens
Grapefruits and grapefruit juice
Halibut
Lactose-free kefir and yogurt
Lactose-free milk
Oranges and orange juice
Potatoes with skin
Salmon
Spinach
Tomatoes

*Q. I'm surprised to see that modified and resistant starches, gums, pectin, and carageenan are allowed? Why is that?*

These food ingredients are a tough call. The terms "modified" and "resistant" starches are non-specific, and include a broad range of starches, including maltodextrin, that can be either naturally present in food or chemically modified. By definition, modified and resistant starches are resistant to digestion in the small intestine and act in a manner similar to fiber in the large intestine, where they are fermented by bacteria and do exert some mild laxative effect. But because they are not short chain molecules (oligo-saccharides), they are fermented more slowly than FODMAPs, and they do not have the same degree of osmotic activity. They fail to meet the definition of FODMAPs, so they are allowed on this diet. Of course, you are free to omit them from your diet if they seem to bother you.

Likewise, gums, pectins and carageenan do not meet the definition of FODMAPs, so they are allowed on this diet. Feel free to omit them from your diet if you wish.

*Q. Why don't you allow spelt on this diet when other sources say it is OK?*

Spelt does have a place in a *low*-FODMAP diet, but to err on the side of caution, I do not allow my clients to have it during the Elimination Phase of the diet. Spelt is another form of wheat. Nutrient analysis of spelt and spelt products has yielded inconsistent numbers for fructan content, possibly having to do with growing conditions, maturity, processing, and cooking. I recognize this is a more conservative approach than you may find elsewhere, but remember the Elimination Phase is only for a couple of weeks. If you find that you do have difficulty with large intakes of fructans, you might, indeed, find that spelt bread products, especially spelt sourdoughs, are easier to digest.

*Q. Where are avocado, beets, broccoli, Brussels sprouts, corn, fennel and pumpkin? They are allowed by some other resources.*

I am aware that by shrinking the portion sizes on these foods it is possible to consume them on a *low*-FODMAP diet. I used the published nutrient data to calculate the FODMAPs in ½ cup portions of these foods. I combined the resulting numbers with my clinical experience and decided to omit these foods from the Elimination Phase of my diet. Even if you discover through the challenge phase that you don't tolerate fructans or polyols very well, you may find that you can include these foods in small portions:

Less than ¼ avocado
Less than ¼ C. beets (beetroot)
Less than ½ C broccoli, Brussels sprouts, sweet corn kernels,
    fennel, or pumpkin

*Q. Why are peanuts allowed? Aren't they a legume?*

Yes, botanically they are a legume, but important enough in the diet to warrant creating a little "fine print" to allow them. Compared to other legumes, peanuts have very little FODMAPs. Also, we tend to eat them in much smaller quantities than other legumes because of their high fat content. For example, 2 T. of peanut butter on a sandwich is a much smaller serving than a two-cup bowlful of bean soup.

*Q. I'm lactose-intolerant, so I don't eat any dairy. Plus, I've always read people with IBS should avoid dairy. Are you sure I should be eating these foods?*

I prefer to the term "milk products" instead of "dairy," thus avoiding the common consumer error of considering eggs a dairy product just because they are sold in the same area of the grocery store. Eggs do not contain lactose.

It is a very common misperception that all milk products are the same when it comes to lactose intolerance, but in fact there is a huge range of lactose in these foods, ranging from none at all in butter and hard cheeses, to about 12 grams for a cup of milk, to almost 30 grams in a cup of canned evaporated milk. Why miss out on all the milk products when you don't have to? Give the lactose-free and very low-lactose milk products a try. You may be pleasantly surprised! Of course, don't try milk products if you have a milk allergy diagnosed by testing, or a history of hives, rash, vomiting, throat swelling, or difficulty breathing after ingesting milk.

*Q. You say that most cheeses and lactose-free milk products are OK, but I have had them in the past and I know I felt bad. What could be going on?*

Please be certain it was the cheese (and not the pizza dough and Coke that went with it) that bothered you in the past. Are you sure it was the lactose-free milk causing symptoms, or was it really the high-fiber breakfast cereal you ate it with? Try to figure this out by using lactose-free milk on the FODMAP Elimination Diet. If it doesn't seem to be bothering you now, then maybe you were mistaken in the past.

If lactose-free milk products still make you feel bad on a low-FODMAP diet, feel free to omit them and find other sources of protein and calcium. Milk and milk products are complicated foods, and IBS is complicated as well. FODMAPs (lactose) aren't the only part of milk products that can cause GI symptoms. Some people are just plain allergic to milk or have another type of sensitivity to it. The way your immune system reacts to milk is affected by the breed of animal the milk is from, what the animals ate, and any heat treatments, fermentation, or processing the milk is subjected to. FODMAPs aren't everything, but following the protocol may at least help you figure out whether you have a lactose problem or problem with milk in general.

*Q. What does lactose-free milk taste like?*

We are trained from childhood, I think, to distrust milk that tastes "off," so many people are reluctant to take a chance on lactose-free milk. Lactose-free milk has a mild, slightly sweeter taste than regular milk, but not enough to be noticeable in tea or on cereal. Drinking it plain allows the sweeter taste to be more apparent, but some of my clients like it just fine; in fact they prefer it!

*Q. I'm lactose-intolerant, but I eat yogurt because they say it is easier to digest. Is that a mistake?*

I don't recommend eating ordinary commercially made yogurt during the Elimination Phase. Traditionally, yogurt was made with raw milk and fermented over an extended period of time—it probably was very low in lactose because the bacteria in the yogurt cultures ate up all the lactose. However, today's commercially prepared yogurt is fermented only briefly, with some thickener such as pectin thrown in to make up for it. Additionally, some commercial yogurts actually have added nonfat dry milk solids or whey that could raise the lactose content significantly. Yogurt makers do not supply information about how many grams of lactose are in their products, so to be on the safe side we assume the worst. All of the "sugar" listed on the food label of plain yogurt could be lactose. If you compare plain yogurt labels, you will see that plain Greek yogurt is probably lower in lactose than other kinds of yogurt.

It is true that many people who are lactose-intolerant can tolerate small portions of regular yogurt, and you may be able have it again in a few weeks. Just don't eat it during the Elimination Phase of this diet.

*Q. I am not lactose-intolerant. Do I still have to use lactose-free milk products?*

I rarely argue with my clients, but I must raise the question: how do you know that you aren't lactose-intolerant? If you had a reliable lactose malabsorption test very recently that you are certain measured both hydrogen and methane gas in your breath, it may be unnecessary to use lactose-free milk products on the Elimination Phase of the diet. However, in my practice I ask almost all my clients to use the lactose-free products during the challenge for the following reasons:

- Most of my clients have never been tested for lactose malabsorption.

- A surprising number of people mistakenly assume they are not lactose-intolerant. They are in for a big surprise when the do the FODMAP Elimination Phase followed by the lactose challenge.

- Even those who do realize they are somewhat lactose-intolerant have numerous misconceptions about the lactose content of foods. For example, many people are under the false impression that unlimited amounts of commercial yogurt are OK on a low-lactose diet.

- False-negative lactose malabsorption breath tests do occur, especially when only breath hydrogen is tested; results of breath tests must be considered together with client history and symptoms.

- If it has been some time since you were tested, you could have developed lactose intolerance since then. It is more common as we get older and can also develop after any gastrointestinal problem that affects the lactase-producing cells lining the small intestine, anything from a bout of gastroenteritis to Crohn's or celiac disease.

- Even adults who tolerate lactose well in general do have limits to how much lactose they can handle. Because the effects of FODMAP carbohydrates are additive, excessive intake of lactose could put you over the top and contribute to symptoms primarily caused by the other FODMAPs.

- Sometimes symptoms following lactose intake are related to rapid transit time caused by other problems. The lactose isn't in the small intestine long enough to be digested and absorbed, even if the person is producing plenty of lactase.

- The Elimination Phase doesn't last forever! If you truly are not lactose intolerant you can return to using regular milk products in just a few weeks.

I recognize that this approach is more conservative than that used by dietitians working in other locales where appropriate breath testing is routine. In my opinion, there is no risk in using lactose-free milk products for a short time, and the potential benefits are vast.

*Q. Why isn't goat's milk allowed? I've read it is better for people with GI problems.*

Goat's milk does have slightly less lactose than cow's milk, but not enough to make a difference for most people. The *proteins* in cow's milk and goat's milk are different enough so that some people with an *allergy* to cow's milk may be able to consume goat's milk, but that is really another subject.

What about that delicious goat cheese that has become so popular? Like cow's milk cheeses, there is less lactose in cheese because most of it is carried off in the whey, which is discarded during the cheese making process. However, un-aged goat cheese probably does have a small amount of lactose in it. It can still be eaten during the Elimination Phase of the diet if the portion is small. Like other non-aged cheeses, the portion of goat cheese should be limited to 1 oz. during the Elimination Phase of the diet. Aged goat cheese, such as cheddar, is allowed.

*Q. Coffee has FODMAPs? How can that be? Please elaborate.*

It does come as a surprise to find fiber in a liquid, but some fibers are soluble in water. According to a study published in 2007, the average 9-ounce "cup" of filtered coffee contains 1.3 grams of fiber. Most of the fiber is a fermentable type and would apparently be defined as FODMAPs in the galactans/GOS category. People who drink three 9-ounce "cups" of coffee a day could be consuming about 4 grams of fiber, equal to the amount in ¾ cup of cooked kidney beans. Who knew?

Many people, including me, would find it very difficult to give up coffee entirely for even a week or two. I suggest, instead, that people undertaking the FODMAP Elimination Diet cut back on coffee to one cup a day. If you are a heavy coffee drinker, cut back on coffee slowly over a week's time before starting the diet to avoid caffeine withdrawal symptoms such as headaches.

If you decide to be a purist, or if your coffee intake is sporadic anyway, then you could completely eliminate coffee. Then, after the Elimination Phase of the diet, you could add decaf coffee back during the galactans/GOS challenge. Challenge with decaf to avoid confusion about the impact of caffeine itself on bowel habits.

*Q. What about herbs, spices, and other seasonings?*

Most herbs, spices, and other seasonings have not been specifically tested for FODMAP composition, but those in the list below can probably be used safely in small amounts. Use more caution with herbs and spices that tend to be used by the teaspoon or tablespoon in recipes, such as ground chili powder, cumin, and cinnamon, until we know more about their FODMAP composition. Use caution with nutmeg, as it can cause nausea and vomiting in large doses.

Baker's yeast
Baking powder
Baking soda/sodium bicarbonate
Black pepper
Chili pepper, red, fresh
Chile or chili powder (100% ground, dried peppers, not chili
    powder blend)
Chives and green (spring) onions, garlic greens—green part only
Cinnamon, ground
Ginger root, fresh or dried
Green leafy herbs, either fresh or dried: parsley, oregano, cilantro,
    dill, marjoram, thyme, rosemary, mint, sage
Paprika
Salt
Seed spices, whole or ground: coriander, mustard, cumin, caraway,
    dill, celery, sesame, poppy, nutmegG
Vanilla extract, real or imitation
Vinegars, except apple cider vinegar

*Q. I'm confused about soy. Is it allowed or isn't it?*

The concern with soy products is the type and amount of carbohydrate (fiber) they contain. Soybean oil, most soy sauces, and lecithin don't contain any carbohydrates, so they are OK for the Elimination Phase of the diet if you see them as ingredients on food labels. Based on their as-yet unpublished data, Australian experts say that tofu is low in FODMAPs. Other soy products, such as soy milk, tempeh, miso, soy protein isolate, and certain imitation meat products, do contain carbohydrates from the soybean, so they are not allowed during the Elimination Phase of the diet.

*Q. Can you go into a little more detail about vinegar? I've read some vinegars are bad for people with GI problems and that unfiltered apple cider vinegar is the best; that's the opposite of what you are saying.*

Remember, this diet is focused on FODMAPs. While most vinegars are low in FODMAPs, a person could still react badly to vinegar for some other reason. Vinegar is complicated. A person could be sensitive to the food the vinegar was made from; vinegars vary in their degree of acidity; aged vinegars like balsamic may contain amines; some stray yeasts can be present in raw vinegars; malt vinegar contains gluten; flavored vinegars may have additives—for example, some commercially seasoned sushi vinegars contain high-fructose corn syrup. All of these factors might influence your ability to tolerate vinegar. Apple cider vinegar is the one vinegar that does contain excess fructose; that is why I do not recommend it on the Elimination Phase of the diet. If you don't tolerate one type of vinegar, try another, or substitute lemon juice in most recipes.

*Q. I keep seeing ads on TV that say high-fructose corn syrup is about the same as regular sugar, so why can't I have it on this diet?*

High-fructose corn syrup does have some similarities to regular sugar. Both provide a similar number of calories per gram. Both contain a mixture of glucose and fructose. Though it is debatable, let's just say for the sake of argument that they are similarly metabolized by your body after they are absorbed.

Our concern is what happens during absorption. Most people absorb fructose reasonably well if it accounts for 50% or less of the sugar in the food. Regular sugar (sucrose) is exactly 50% fructose, every time.

What the ads aren't telling you is that different versions of high-fructose corn syrups are used in different products, and you can't tell which one you are about to consume by reading the food label. The fructose content of popular sugar-sweetened beverages is nearly always higher than 55%; some popular colas are 65% fructose. While that might look to some people as if it is "about the same" as sugar, your body can tell the difference. High-fructose corn syrup is therefore not allowed on the Elimination Phase of the diet.

Just to complicate matters a little bit further, ordinary corn syrup is almost 100% dextrose (glucose) so it is allowed on the Elimination Phase of the diet.

*Q. Why isn't agave syrup allowed? It's meant to be a healthy alternative to sugar.*

Despite its reputation as a natural sweetener, agave syrup is actually highly processed. Up to 90% of the sugars in agave syrup are fructose, and that clearly marks it as high in FODMAPs.

*Q. I am on the go all the time and usually eat a lot of pre-packaged fiber, fruit, protein, or snack bars. What can I do now?*

Your previous high intake of these bars might have been causing you a lot of grief, as they tend to be loaded with FODMAPs. These are perfect examples of hard-to-digest foods that were not in our food supply in years past, since the first granola bars didn't come on the market in the U.S. until 1975! If you find you are fructose, fructan, or galactan sensitive, you will eventually need to find other solutions for eating on the run. For now, try the recipe for Pecan Pie Granola Bars in this book to fill that niche in your diet. In a pinch, you could use classic Nature Valley Crunchy Granola Bars (peanut butter, roasted almond, or cinnamon), which are still made without high-fructose corn syrup, sugar alcohols, or new-fangled fiber or protein ingredients. They contain soy flour as an ingredient, so aren't a perfect match for the Elimination Phase, but they come as close as any commercial bar I have seen to being low in FODMAPs.

*Q. I can't believe gluten is allowed on this diet. Isn't gluten bad for people with gut problems? How can I trust the rest of your advice you if you allow gluten?*

Some people take it as an article of faith that gluten grains are bad for everyone, and that we are all ruining our health by eating them. I don't share that opinion; I think it is an overgeneralization. Don't miss this important point: this diet is narrowly focused on eliminating FODMAPs. Gluten is not a FODMAP, so it is allowed if you do not have celiac disease. Of course, gluten is bad for some people with gut problems, but the whole point of this program is to get away from one-size-fits-all diets. You can trust me to be sensible, to teach you how to think logically about how your food affects you, and to help you apply the latest research to your everyday life in the twenty-first century. I respect your skepticism, however. You definitely should think critically about this or any other diet. Health and nutrition experts have different world views, and you need to find a solution that matches your values. You should eat and feed your family the best you can with the time and money you have available, not feel guilty or ashamed if you fall short of someone else's idealistic vision of dietary perfection.

*Q. How can I evaluate the information on the Nutrition Facts panel to figure out whether I can eat a food?*

You can sometimes use the Nutrition Facts panel on a food package to figure out whether or not something has FODMAPs in it. Let's use Kikkoman Soy Sauce as an example. The first place to check is the list of ingredients at the bottom of the panel. If the product has added sugars, fibers, or polyols, or food ingredients that contain them, you will see them listed. This sauce contains water, wheat, soybeans, salt, and sodium benzoate. Hmm. Suspicion is raised because it contains soy and wheat. Because of the wheat, this is not a gluten-free product, so not appropriate for those with celiac disease or gluten sensitivity, but does it really contain FODMAPs?

The next place to check is total carbohydrates per serving. All FODMAPs, by definition, are carbohydrates. "Total carbohydrates" on the Nutrition Facts Panel is the sum of the sugars, fibers, sugar alcohols, and "other" carbohydrates (usually starches). If the total carbohydrates are zero, then one serving of the product is likely to be fine to eat on the FODMAP Elimination Diet.

- Lactose and fructose will show up on the nutrition facts as "sugars."
- Fructans and galactans/GOS will show up on the nutrition facts as "fiber."
- Polyols (sugar alcohols) are harder to spot. If the product makes a claim on the label about sugar, and sugar alcohols are present in the food, they must be listed on a separate line. If not, they are lumped in with "other carbohydrates," which are often not listed on the food label at all. How can we make an educated guess whether or not this food might contain polyols? Polyols enter our diet as natural components of certain fruits, vegetables, and sweeteners added to food. Let's have one more look at the ingredients. There are no added sweeteners and no fruit or vegetable ingredients, so probably no polyols.

In our example, the total carbohydrates listed on the food label are "zero." One serving of this food probably contains little or no FODMAPs. It is a safe bet that this brand of soy sauce can be eaten during the Elimination Phase of the FODMAP diet. You can use the same reasoning for other foods.

*Q. One of my medications contains glycerin, lactose, or another ingredient that is "not allowed." What should I do?*

You should continue taking your medication as prescribed. You should never discontinue a medication without first discussing it with the prescribing provider. Don't stress over this for the short term of the Elimination Phase of the diet. If your symptoms are triggered by FODMAPs, the change in diet alone should give you as much information as you need. If you learn through the challenge process that you are particularly sensitive to a type of FODMAP you are consuming regularly in your medication, you can discuss alternatives on a case-by-case basis with your pharmacist and the prescribing provider.

Some medications do contain "inactive ingredients" that are FODMAPs, but the amounts are generally very small. Glycerin, also known as glycerine or glycerol, is a polyol and a potential laxative taken in quantity. It is sometimes used in very small amounts in supplements or pharmaceuticals for its properties as a lubricant and a moisturizer. When it comes to FODMAPs, the quantity ingested is critical. The amount of polyols in 100 grams of mushrooms is 2.74 grams. That is about 200 times more than the miniscule amount of glycerine in 2 capsules of one probiotic supplement on the market. The small amount present in such a supplement wouldn't be likely to cause a problem.

Lactose is likely to be present in larger amounts; individuals who are exquisitely sensitive to lactose and take large numbers of pills, tablets, or capsules may wish to take a serious look at how many grams of lactose per day they are ingesting through medications.

*Q. What should I look for in a multi-vitamin with minerals supplement*

- No food or plant-based ingredients. If you suspect you have food intolerances, you are asking for trouble with these
- A capsule with powder inside, a powder, a chewable, or a liquid to maximize absorption in case of rapid transit time or poor digestion
- Two per day dosing will improve the rate of nutrient absorption
- Very little to no calcium, magnesium, or iron to minimize GI side effects (take separately if indicated). Vitamin C is OK, but not in excess

- Not much more than 100% of DV for most nutrients unless treating a specific deficiency (except perhaps vitamin B-12)
- Doesn't cost an arm and a leg
- Doesn't require taking handfuls of capsules per day
- Folate in the form of L-methyl folate
- No lactose, fructose, or sugar alcohols as sweeteners

*Q. I have lost some weight while on the Elimination Phase of the diet. Is that OK?*

Weight loss might be perfectly appropriate for some people, but not for others. The answer to this question is so individual in nature that you must discuss it with the health care provider who knows you best. Don't put this off if you are underweight to begin with or feeling concerned about your weight.

*Q. I am working with a dietitian. When is the best time to schedule a follow up appointment?*

I recommend seeing your dietitian again three weeks after the initial appointment. That gives you a week to eat up your "old" groceries, buy new ones, and get ready, and two weeks to execute the Elimination Phase of the diet. At your second visit, your dietitian can help you review the results of the Elimination Phase of the diet and plan what you will eat and drink during the Challenge Phase.

*Q. The Elimination Phase is working a little too well! Even though I have diarrhea-predominant IBS, I am actually feeling a little constipated on the Elimination Phase. What should I do?*

This is a good time to review basic constipation prevention measures, which you have probably never had to worry about before now.

- Increase your water consumption. This area might need extra attention if you were previously drinking a lot of coffee, fruit juice, or regular soft drinks. Your body might be missing those fluids, even if it is not missing the FODMAPs!
- Increase your activity level. Even some light walking after meals may help. Consult your physician before sharply increasing the amount or intensity of exercise.
- Eat higher fiber choices from the allowed grains and starches, such as oatmeal/porridge, oat bran, winter squash,

brown rice, rice bran, quinoa, corn pasta, and potatoes with the skin.

- Try larger portions of the allowed vegetables.

*Q. Where did you get the data used to rank the lactose content of these foods?*

It would be very helpful if producers of milk products would report the number of grams of lactose in their products to consumers, but that is not the case. Maybe the facts would interfere with the popular notion that yogurt is "easier to digest" than milk. When I can't find facts about the lactose content of milk products, I have to estimate it using the "total sugars" reported on the Nutrition Facts panel or in the USDA Nutrient Database for Standard Reference. In milk products with no added sugar, it is logical that the amount of lactose cannot exceed the total sugars. I recognize that fermented milk products have had some of the lactose consumed by the live cultures in the products, so the lactose content is probably somewhat less than the total sugars.

*Q. Is there a way to distinguish lactose intolerance from casein sensitivity during the Challenge Phase?*

If even the lactose-free milk products on the allowed food lists make you feel unwell, then your problem with milk goes beyond lactose. It could be a problem with the protein in the milk (casein) or some other aspect of the milk such as the way it was processed, the mammal species that produced the milk (cow, goat, buffalo, sheep, camel) or the feed the animal ate.

*Q. I already know I am lactose-intolerant—do I have to do that challenge?*

You don't absolutely have to do it, if you don't want to, of course. But I can tell you that I have had more than one patient who made that faulty assumption and found out during the lactose challenge that they actually were not lactose-intolerant after all.

*Q. The ranking order of the foods in the fructans category seems off. I've read that garlic has more fructans than any other food, but you've ranked it toward the bottom of the list. What gives?*

Nutrient composition tables usually show the grams of fructans per 100 grams of the food. No one eats 100 grams (over 3 ounces) of garlic at one sitting. A clove of garlic weighs about 3 grams, so when we compare a one clove serving of garlic to a bowl of high-fiber breakfast cereal, it contains much less fructans.

*Q. Why is sourdough bread listed lower than other breads?*

Some recent published data demonstrates the fructan content in spelt sourdough bread is quite low. Authentic sourdough bread uses a lactobacillus and wild yeast starter instead of baker's yeast, and it ferments during a longer rising period. Possibly microorganisms in the sourdough culture "pre-digest" some of the fructans that would otherwise be present in the bread. Speak to your baker to make sure no baker's yeast is added to speed up the rise.

*Q. If I react badly to wheat products, is there a way to distinguish non-celiac gluten intolerance from fructans intolerance during the Challenge Phase?*

I think this is an important question because gluten-free eating has become a popular choice, even for people who do not have celiac disease or non-celiac gluten sensitivity. Eating a gluten-free diet when you don't really have to is an unnecessary burden. It makes it more difficult for you to participate in family events, eat in restaurants, shop, and cook. The food is more expensive. The diet is less varied, which is undesirable from a nutrition standpoint unless absolutely necessary. A gluten challenge may be called for to try and figure whether a gluten-free diet is necessary for you. Obviously, if you have a confirmed diagnosis of celiac disease, you should not challenge yourself with gluten. I would also not recommend a gluten challenge without medical supervision if your suspected gluten-related symptoms last more than a day, occur with even the most minimal intake of gluten, or are not limited to IBS (for example headache, rash, sinusitis, or achy joints).

If you do still occasionally eat foods containing gluten and have gut-only symptoms that are clearly evident following a "dietary indiscretion," you could try eating pure gluten to see what happens. Do this after you have completed the Challenge Phase of the FODMAP diet. The purpose would be to figure out whether gluten is causing your GI symptoms or if it is some other aspect of the wheat. Gluten is one of the proteins found in wheat, rye, and barley. In some cuisines, it is isolated from the wheat, processed, and made into a high-protein food called seitan. Vital wheat gluten is also used in bread baking to improve the texture, elasticity, and rise of the bread. Therefore, it can usually be purchased in the baking aisle of any well-stocked grocery store. Look for a brand of vital wheat gluten that has zero grams of fiber and zero grams of sugar per serving, therefore, no FODMAPs.

There are many creative ways to make seitan from scratch and then utilize it as a meat substitute in recipes. However, for the purpose at hand I recommend a simple recipe with few other ingredients, such as the one that follows this chapter. Eat a full serving of seitan a couple of times and monitor your symptoms. If there are none, then you should discuss with your dietitian or health care provider whether it is really necessary for you to follow a gluten-free diet for your gastrointestinal symptoms. In addition, because symptoms of gluten intolerance can sometimes be delayed, you should remain alert for the reappearance of symptoms after you have been eating gluten again for a longer period of time.

*Q. I was fine when I challenged with fructans. What's the harm in eating bread while I do the rest of the challenges?*

The FODMAP effect is cumulative. If your bucket is half full of fructans from bread, it is stacking the deck against the next group of FODMAPs you are challenging. Wait just a little longer; you will be back to eating bread in no time. It will be worth the extra effort to work around bread for the better quality information you will get from the rest of the challenges.

*Q. How long does it take for symptoms to appear after eating an offending food? What is the significance of the timing?*

The time frame for symptoms to develop after eating FODMAPs ranges from hours to days. FODMAPs don't exert their effects until they have traveled through your system to the far end of the small intestine and into the large intestine. This "intestinal transit time" varies from person to person, and can vary based on the presence of inflammation or illness in the intestines and the composition of the diet. At the far end of the time frame, once the FODMAPs have been eliminated from your body in the feces, their effects are over.

Here is a "before" example of this effect: John has frequent early morning diarrhea and must get up early to use the toilet repeatedly before work. He then feels "safe" to go to work but doesn't dare eat much during the day lest he have a bout of his IBS symptoms. In the evening, of course, he is starving and loads up on a day's worth of food and FODMAPs in just a few hours. Not surprisingly, by morning, poorly digested or absorbed carbohydrates have traveled to his large intestine, and he is symptomatic again. A vicious cycle has been perpetuated.

Here is an "after" example: Jean is on the elimination diet. Everything she eats is low- FODMAP except for her lactose challenge. By the end of the challenge day, after several servings of regular milk products, Jean is feeling bloated, gassy, and a little nauseous. In the morning, she has several bouts of watery diarrhea. She returns to the Elimination Phase of the diet, consumes no more lactose, and feels better by evening.

If your symptoms occur immediately after eating, they are less likely to be due to FODMAPs. The one exception would be the scenario in which the large intestine is full of gas from an earlier meal and is exerting upward pressure on the stomach. New food of any kind entering the stomach might then cause uncomfortable feelings of fullness, bloating, or even some gastroesophageal reflux.

If your symptoms linger for days, long after you have eliminated the remnants of the suspect food, they are less likely to be due to FODMAPs. For example, a woman doing the fructans challenge eats a piece of regular bread on Monday and becomes symptomatic. She does not continue with the fructans challenge and returns to the Elimination Phase of the diet, but she is still recovering from eating the piece of bread on Thursday. This woman should raise the subject with her physician and discuss testing for other types of adverse reactions to wheat.

*Q. I ate one piece of bread for my "cautious" fructans challenge. Boy, was I sick! What should I do next?*

Repeat the cautious challenge with another wheat or rye product and do not advance to the more aggressive challenge. If the bad experience is repeated, it raises the possibility of undiagnosed celiac disease or non-celiac gluten sensitivity which should be explored with your health care provider. You could consider doing the fructans challenge another time using only the vegetables on the fructans list.

*Q. I challenged a particular group of FODMAPs and I had no symptoms. Can I go back to eating them now?*

That's great news! You should continue to leave them out of your diet until you are finished with all the challenges, but after that you can start eating them again.

For example, if your body produces plenty of the enzyme lactase, you won't have trouble digesting lactose (milk sugar). If you challenge yourself with several generous helpings of regular milk products and experience no increase in gas, bloating, abdominal pain, or diarrhea, you are free to enjoy milk products any time with no restrictions.

*Q. I challenged a particular group of FODMAPs and my symptoms were severe. How can I cope with that?*

If you do have uncomfortable symptoms when challenging yourself, you will have learned something very important for your troubles. Knowledge is power! The results of this process are subjective, and you are the judge. You decide whether these are symptoms you can live with. There are a variety of ways to handle this situation. There may be some FODMAP foods that you choose to permanently drop from your diet, but that isn't always necessary.

The challenge food lists are ranked in roughly descending order. Foods at the bottom of each list have the least FODMAPs. You can use this information to guide your food choices. For example, let's say you find you are highly intolerant of polyols. You know that polyol-sweetened candy is something that you will happily just avoid from now on. You may find that you can still enjoy small portions of foods selected from the bottom of that list.

Here is another example that demonstrates the portion control strategy. Let's say you got severe symptoms from your galactans/GOS challenge. One cup of your grandmother's baked beans potentially has 16 times more galactans/GOS in it than a tablespoon of beanson your salad, just because it has 16 times more beans! Give yourself a chance to try enjoying small portions of high-FODMAP foods before you write them off altogether.

*Q. I was kind of uncomfortable during one of the challenges, but it really wasn't too bad. Should I re-challenge it?*

Make sure that you chose foods from the top of the challenge list (most FODMAPs) and that you had several large portions. If you were too tentative or cautious, try again. If you gave it a good challenge the first time, there is no need to repeat it.

This situation will be relatively easy to manage. When you choose to eat that type of FODMAP, choose foods from lower on the FODMAP list and eat small or medium portions. Limit other FODMAPs in the same meal or day. For example, you may be able eat a few tablespoons of beans in a soup or salad, but not a cup of refried beans. If you do have a cup of beans, don't wash it down with a Coke or a milkshake.

Don't lose sight of the fact that consistently filling up your bucket half-way with these foods can still contribute significantly to overflowing symptoms on high-FODMAP days. Keep an eye on them. In my experience, fructans are particularly likely to cause trouble in this way, since our food supply in the U.S. is so wheat-heavy.

*Q. If I react badly to one food within a group, should I assume that I can't tolerate all the other foods in that group. For example, if I can't tolerate bagels, does that mean I need to avoid all the foods in the fructan group?*

No. Remember, we are trying to assess tolerance to a type of carbohydrate in our diet rather than our tolerance to individual foods. It's important not to over-generalize, because it is a nutritional mistake to unnecessarily restrict your diet. Please discuss this sort of question with your dietitian before jumping to conclusions that would lead you to permanently restrict any large group of foods.

For example, there are a number of things that could explain a bad reaction to one food in a group without warranting generalization to the rest of the group:

- You might be allergic to that food
- You might have celiac disease or non-celiac gluten intolerance but be fine with vegetable sources of fructans
- Other foods in the same group might have much less fructans per serving than the one that bothers you
- Your portion size of other foods in that group might be much smaller
- The specific type of fructans in the food might be more or less rapidly fermentable than others

*Q. I feel a lot better, but I still have some gas. How can I get rid of it?*

It is normal and healthy to have some gas, as long as you are not in pain, so you probably shouldn't worry. Bacterial fermentation of carbohydrates in the gut is a necessary and normal process that provides important health benefits. The average person produces several pints of gas a day and might pass gas up to a dozen times per day. In fact, passing some gas as flatulence might reduce your pain from bloating. OK, so it can be socially unacceptable to pass gas in some situations. Come up with an excuse to take a quick walk to the parking lot or around the block and let some of that gas go! Avoid tight waistbands so that your abdominal wall can relax and expand a little bit as needed.

*Q. The diet didn't work for me at all. What can I take away from this experience?*

It is a fact that for some individuals, IBS symptoms may not be triggered by FODMAP carbohydrate malabsorption. Even this information can be a valuable outcome of the elimination diet. You'll be free to enjoy foods, knowing that they are probably not IBS triggers for you, at least not because they contain FODMAPs.

Note that some scientists and clinicians have found that foods can trigger IBS symptoms in certain individuals by another mechanism: delayed immune response. A very effective program for identifying and treating this type of adverse food reaction has been developed. It is called LEAP therapy. LEAP® stands for Lifestyle Eating and Performance. Signet Diagnostic Corporation developed Mediator Release Testing (MRT®) which is a blood test for sensitivity to a large panel of foods and food chemicals. A detailed, customized elimination diet is then planned for each patient based on the results of the test. Specially trained dietitians (Certified LEAP Therapists or CLTs) work with patients throughout the program. Although further discussion of LEAP is outside the scope of this book, I encourage you to look into it if you live in the U.S., particularly if you have other, difficult-to-treat inflammatory conditions in addition to IBS, such as migraine headache, chronic sinusitis, or fibromyalgia.

*Q. Friday pizza night with the family is very important to me and I don't want to give it up, even though too many fructans make me feel crummy. How can I manage this?*

There may be times when you are willing to experience some discomfort in order to enjoy something special, such as pizza night or a summer picnic with watermelon and sweet corn. That's perfectly OK.

Planning ahead is the best strategy to use for eating events you know about in advance. For example, if you know you are going to have pizza for dinner, choose not to have a bagel for breakfast or an onion and pepper fajita for lunch! Remember, other FODMAPs help fill up the bucket, too. Pull out your elimination diet materials and plan low-FODMAP meals and snacks for the rest of the day. Leave lots of room in your bucket for the pizza. Think about ways to manage the portion of the pizza dough—thin crust pizza makes a big difference. Or get a smaller sized pizza and add a side salad.

*Q. Since I've been on this diet, it seems like I am having a problem with a particular food that isn't even high in FODMAPs. Why am I noticing this now?*

If all goes well, you will have dramatically fewer IBS symptoms within a week or two on the Elimination Phase of this diet. This can sometimes make other types of adverse food reactions "pop out" at you. Perhaps you've heard of the "blackboard" analogy. When the blackboard is smeared with chalk and full of scribbles, it's hard to make out any one particular mark. But when it has been thoroughly cleaned with a damp cloth, it is possible to clearly see even a small mark on the board from the back of the room. For example, I had a client with chronic constipation who became aware in the course of the FODMAP Elimination Diet that every time he ate eggs for breakfast, his constipation got worse. Since eggs don't contain FODMAPs, this was a completely incidental discovery, but one he was happy to have made.

*Q. Are there any absolutely prohibited foods after the Challenge Phase?*

No. That is the whole point of this program. You can eat any foods that you tolerate, in the amounts that work for you.

*Q. What if I fail all the FODMAP challenges?*

You may have to build your meal plans more closely around the foods allowed on the elimination diet than other people, and use all of the strategies for individual FODMAPs that are discussed below. However, there are a few other ideas worth considering.

Is there any reason that your belly cannot gently expand to accommodate the four pints or so of gas you product each day? For example, have you gained weight but continued to wear your old clothes with tight waistbands?

Have you had abdominal surgery that has changed your anatomy? For example, one of my clients had a particular type of breast re-construction surgery (after a double mastectomy) that involved pulling up her abdominal wall and reinforcing it with a rigid mesh panel. The slightest increase in gas production was causing her abdominal pain because there was no place for that gas to go. Reducing her overall FODMAP load helped a lot.

If all the FODMAP foods trigger your gas and bloating symptoms, it may be that your intestinal transit time is just too fast due an underlying infection or disease process. You may be experiencing a "freight train effect" which is rushing the sugars and sugar alcohols through the tunnel so fast they can't be properly digested and absorbed. If you haven't already, I would encourage you to seek evaluation by a gastroenterologist.

If you are experiencing alternating diarrhea and constipation worsened by FODMAPs, pay special attention to consistency in your meal patterns and food choices. It's unrealistic to expect your body to somehow produce a perfectly formed, on-time stool every day when you are sporadic and inconsistent in its care and feeding. Feed yourself a little bit more like you feed your pet dog or cat—a consistent diet on a regular schedule. Yes, variety is important, but you can add variety within a consistent meal pattern or framework.

Be certain that you aren't over-treating episodes of constipation with laxatives, stool softeners, fiber supplements, and high-fiber foods, which will empty you out, cause a delay in your next bowel movement that is perceived as constipation, and perpetuate the cycle. If you still need these products in addition to your low-FODMAP diet, work with your health care provider to establish a constipation prevention care plan, perhaps using a fraction of a dose of such a product daily, rather than waiting to treat constipation after it has occurred.

*Q. Will my FODMAP intolerance ever get better, or am I stuck with this problem for life?*

FODMAP intolerance can be temporary if is occurring during an episode of an underlying disease process. For example, it is common for patients with untreated celiac disease, a flare-up of Crohn's disease, or recovering from a bad bout of gastroenteritis to experience lactose intolerance. The cells lining the small intestine may be temporarily impaired in their ability to produce lactase. When the small intestine heals, lactase production can resume, and lactose intolerance eases. Any condition that speeds up your intestinal transit time can cause a secondary FODMAP intolerance that could clear up or improve as the underlying condition improves.

With regard to fructans and galactans/GOS, many experts believe that the bowels can adapt to very gradually increased intake of these fibers. It is to your benefit to consume these fibers if you can tolerate them. Start with small servings of the foods at the bottom of the challenge lists and work your way up.

*Q. It appears I am lactose-intolerant. Should I just quit drinking milk?*

No. Milk and milk products are important sources of protein, vitamins, and minerals in the diet, and they taste good, too! Rice or almond milk can't really take the place of milk nutritionally, because they contain very little protein.

Many people with lactose malabsorption find they can actually tolerate small amounts of lactose, so it is rarely necessary to be on a lactose-free diet. A low-lactose diet will be enough to manage symptoms for all but the most sensitive individuals.

If you discover that you need to limit your lactose consumption, continue to use lactose-free milk, cottage cheese, yogurt, kefir, and ice cream at home as you did during the Elimination Phase, and carry some lactase pills with you in case you find yourself eating ice cream or chowder away from home. When selecting a lactase product, read the label carefully. Unbelievably, some lactase supplements contain mannitol, a polyol.

Commercial lactose-free milk products are treated with the lactase enzyme before they are packaged, to break milk down sugar (lactose) into smaller units that can be absorbed. Mixing is thorough and complete before the product is packaged, and the product is rendered 100% lactose-free. When you take a lactase pill, the mixing is not as thorough and complete in your body as it is at the dairy plant! The pill may knock the grams of lactose in the product down to a tolerable level, but it will not render it lactose-free.

*Q. I've heard that some medications contain lactose. If I'm lactose-intolerant, what should I do about this?*

It's true: lactose is the most common filler used in the manufacture of drugs. While the amount of lactose per pill might be small, people who are on multiple medications or must take large numbers of pills could be consuming several grams of lactose per day in this way.

If you are concerned about this, you can ask your pharmacist how much lactose is in your medications. Lactose-free alternatives are often available. Do not stop taking or change a medication before discussing it with the health care provider who prescribed it.

*Q. Fructose was the worst one for me. Is there anything equivalent to lactase tablets that will help me digest fructose?*

Fructose doesn't need digesting. It is already the smallest possible sugar unit and is absorbed "as is." People with fructose malabsorption just absorb fructose too slowly. You can't take a pill for that, but there are some other strategies you can use.

Polyols seem to make fructose absorption worse, so you can help yourself by avoiding fruits that have both excess fructose and polyols.

You can also consider eating some extra glucose (also known as dextrose) with higher-fructose fruits, which seems to sweep along some fructose as it is absorbed. You can buy glucose (dextrose) powder at supplement shops, beer and wine-making suppliers, or on the Internet, and experiment with it. Glucose (dextrose) tablets are sold at the local pharmacy for diabetics who need to give their blood sugar a boost. This strategy only works if fructose is the only FODMAP present in the food.

Some patients report their tolerance for fruit improves when it is part of a smoothie containing protein powder. This could be due to the fact that amino acids, the building blocks of protein, may enhance fructose absorption, possibly by sweeping some fructose along as it is absorbed.

Fructosin® is a new enzyme supplement on the market in Europe. It contains the enzyme xylose isomerase. This is not a digestive enzyme like lactase. Its primary industrial use is just the opposite, converting glucose to fructose in the production of high-fructose corn syrup. However, the manufacturer claims that Fructosin will convert fructose to glucose when taken with food, thereby reducing the fructose load of the meal and fructose malabsorption. If these claims prove true, this could someday be a helpful supplement for use with high-fructose foods; however, its effectiveness hasn't yet been established.

*Q. I have trouble with fructans. Any special tips for me?*

In the U.S., wheat provides the vast majority of fructans in the diet. Cut back on your consumption of wheat products overall. Locate a source of artisan sourdough wheat or sourdough spelt bread. Authentic sourdough breads are allowed to ferment over a longer time period while rising than breads to which baker's yeast is added. The longer fermentation time may allow the microbes in the sourdough culture to break down some of the fructans. Check the label—if baker's yeast is added to speed up the rise, the sourdough bread will not be as good for your purposes.

Cook with garlic-infused oil instead of garlic. Cook with big chunks of garlic or onion and take them out of the food before you eat it. Start an herb garden and grow some chives. Experiment with other leafy herbs and sweet spices.

Try to get your fiber from intact foods and skip the isolated fibers added as ingredients. These ingredients may help food companies market their products as "high-fiber," but they don't do anything to help you if fructans trigger your IBS symptoms.

*Q. What about an enzyme to break down fructans?*

It seems to me that such an enzyme might be of limited value; it would release a flood of free fructose into the gut, with no net decrease in the FODMAP load, perhaps worsening the plight of people with fructose malabsorption. However, certain individuals may absorb fructose well but not tolerate fructans; they might benefit from experimenting with enzymes.

*Q. Can I work around the fructans problem by eating gluten-free bread and pizza dough?*

You are welcome to give it a try, but one recent study in the United Kingdom showed that some gluten-free products contain just as many fructans as regular breads.

Also, many gluten-free breads and baked goods include substantial amounts of xanthan gum as an ingredient. Xanthan gum, which does not meet the strict definition of a FODMAP, shares certain characteristics with FODMAPs and is poorly tolerated by some individuals. DeLand Bakery has a very tasty line of wheat-free (not gluten-free) breads made without xanthan gum. DeLand products are available at Whole Foods and at independent health food stores.

If you are not gluten-intolerant, spelt or sourdough spelt products might be the answer. Or you may have to focus on filling the "carbohydrate" slot in your lunch box or dinner plate with alternative whole grains and starchy vegetables rather than bread. Look to ethnic cuisines that rely more on rice, corn products, oats, millet, quinoa, or potatoes for inspiration.

*Q. If I have fructose malabsorption, do I automatically have to limit fructans as well, since fructans are chains of fructose molecules linked together?*

Not necessarily. It is a mistake to over-generalize that everyone with dietary fructose intolerance (aka FM) automatically cannot tolerate other FODMAPs. The fact that fructans consist of fructose chains isn't particularly significant, since humans don't have the enzymes to break these bonds and liberate the fructose molecules. Fructans can be poorly tolerated in their own right, due their fermentability and osmotic activity. It is true that some people with fructose malabsorption also poorly tolerate fructans or other FODMAPs, making the FODMAP elimination and challenge process worthwhile for those with a diagnosis of fructose malabsorption.

*Q. Those polyols killed me. Is there any help for that?*

Not much. There is one study that shows amino acid (in a protein powder, for example) might help enhance sorbitol absorption, but that isn't of much practical value for dealing with the polyols in most foods.

Eat small servings of candy made with real sugar. Ask your mother what kind of gum she chewed in 1970 and get some old-fashioned, sugar-sweetened gum.

Avoid bingeing when high-polyol fruits and vegetables are in season. You may learn in time that small daily portions of mushrooms or dates actually help you stay regular, but that eating quarts of cherries or bushels of apples when they are in season is a bad idea.

*Q. Are there any specific tips for people who don't tolerate galactans/GOS?*

To reduce the FODMAP content of beans, lentils, or split peas, be sure to soak them for 3-12 hours before cooking, drain, add fresh water for cooking, and discard the cooking water. If the beans are canned, drain, soak and rinse them before using. Don't make the mistake I made, thinking that the thick liquid in the can of beans would make a nice rich broth for my chili!

Some studies have shown that naturally fermented beans and bean flours are significantly lower in galactans/GOS, so you could experiment with tempeh, fermented beans pastes such as miso, fermented black beans such as nattō, and so on.

Sprouting legumes (pulses) is reputed to reduce their galactan content, but the sprouting process can encourage the growth of bacteria that cause food-borne illness. To be on the safe side, cook all sprouted legumes to 165° F.

The enzyme alpha-galactosidase, found in some over-the-counter enzyme products such as Beano® and Digest Spectrum®, is reported to break galacatans/GOS apart into galactose molecules which can be absorbed by humans. This enzyme should be used with caution by people with galactosemia or diabetes. It is derived from aspergillis niger, so it should not be used by people with allergy or sensitivity to molds.

*Q. I don't eat meat. How should I manage that, given the high-FODMAP content of legumes (pulses), which I rely on for protein?*

Work with a registered dietitian, if possible, to make sure your nutrient intake is adequate. Keep the Elimination Phase as short as possible, no more than one or two weeks. Lean on tofu and quinoa for protein. After the Challenge Phase, adding other soy products, lentils, and beans gradually, as tolerated, will help meet your daily requirement for protein. Start with the foods at the bottom of the challenge list which contain less galactans/GOS. Eat your legumes in small, frequent meals rather than one large evening meal. Because these foods are such an important part of the vegetarian diet, you may choose to eat most of your FODMAPs in this form. Keep your bucket from filling up by choosing lower FODMAP fruits and vegetables, limiting the amount of wheat products in your diet, and continuing to use lactose-free milk products if lactose-intolerant.

*Q. I am looking at a food label and everything looks OK except for that one joy-killer there toward the end of the ingredients list. Can I eat this food?*

During the Elimination Phase, the answer would be "no"—you were trying to be a purist, then. But now, the answer is a distinct…maybe.

The first thing to know is that ingredients are listed on food labels in descending order, by weight. That means that the items toward the end of the list are present in ever smaller amounts. Your level of tolerance for that particular type of FODMAP will also influence your decision. If you have severe fructose malabsorption, you probably won't want a granola bar with high-fructose corn syrup as the first ingredient, but if it is at the end of a list in a cracker or something that is clearly not all that sweet, it might be fine.

*Q. What are probiotics and should I take them?*

When we restrict FODMAPs, we deprive gut bacteria of their favorite foods. This decreases gas and bloating symptoms. But we don't want to give up the benefits of having a healthy number and balance of "good" bacteria in our guts. Taking probiotic supplements can help us navigate this tricky situation. Probiotics are microbes (usually bacteria) that we deliberately ingest in doses that are large enough to have a medicinal effect.

People with IBS (and eating a FODMAP-restricted diet) need a gut stocked with critters that are happy with a diet of non-FODMAP carbohydrates, ***don't*** produce excessive gas, and ***do*** produce large amounts of desirable, healthy substances called short chain fatty acids. Probiotics influence gut pH, help the immune system function properly, and diminish the influence of bad bacteria. There is emerging clinical evidence that probiotics may reduce visceral hypersensitivity, the tendency to feel gut sensations as painful. Probiotics known as Bifidobacteria, Lactobacillus plantarum (Lp299v), Lactobacillus GG and Saccharomyces boulardii are all good candidates.

If you are already using a probiotic before you start the FODMAP Elimination Diet, you should continue to use it throughout the process.

If you are not already using a probiotic, it is probably best to wait until after the Challenge Phase to start taking one. At the very least, I'd suggest removing the fermentable carbs from your diet before you start one; in other words, wait until you have completed the Elimination Phase. When you decide to add a probiotic, consider the following tips:

- Consider choosing a probiotic product including one or more of the following: Bifidobacteria (especially B. infantis), Lactobacillus plantarum (Lp299v), or Lactobacillus GG.

- Individuals with antibiotic-associated or post-infectious IBS with diarrhea might benefit also from Saccharomyces boulardii, which is different from most probiotics because it is a yeast, not a bacteria.

- Purchase your probiotics from a retailer that cares about temperature-controlled storage and shipping. Although some products are now shelf-stable and don't necessarily have to be refrigerated at all times, their potency can still be diminished by extended storage at temperatures over 70° F.

- Don't kill the good bacteria in your probiotic product by taking it with hot coffee or hot oatmeal! Take your probiotics with a cold meal or well before or after a hot meal or drink.

- If you tend to be very sensitive to changes in your health regimen, open the probiotic capsule and begin with just a fraction of a dose sprinkled on some cold food or stirred into a cool glass of water. Work your way up to the full labeled dose over a few days time.

- Probiotics have a sort of threshold effect. You won't get the full medicinal effect  the product was intended, designed, and tested for if you don't take a big enough dose, so don't skimp. Because probiotics don't seem to linger or colonize in the gut, you should take them on a regular basis.

- Even if you don't usually take probiotics, consider using them following a bout of food poisoning, gastroenteritis, or antibiotic use.

- If your immune system is compromised due to illness or immune-suppressing drugs, discuss the risks and benefits with your health care provider before using probiotics.

- During the FODMAP Elimination Diet, or if you do not wish to take probiotic supplements, you can get probiotics from lactose-free yogurt or kefir with *live* cultures.

## *Conclusion*

Congratulations! I hope that the end of this diet protocol marks the beginning of a brilliant new chapter in your life. May the knowledge you have earned help you be IBS-free at last. May you take fearless pleasure in eating delicious and nutritious food. I hope your experience of health and well-being will allow you new freedom to reach your other life goals. Please visit www.ibsfree.net to share your comments and experiences with me and with your fellow travelers on this journey. We can continue learning from each other.

# A FEW BASIC RECIPES

*IBS—Free at Last!* is not meant to be a cookbook. It is meant to teach you a way to think about your food and how it may be affecting your symptoms. Most people have their hands full during the Elimination Phase of the diet with label reading, planning, and preparing very simple meals. Still, there are a few simple recipes that may make the FODMAP Elimination Diet easier and tastier, and I offer them here.

## Garlic-Infused Oil

Get the irreplaceable flavor of garlic without the stomach ache. Use garlic-infused oil as a cooking or flavoring oil.

½ C. extra-virgin olive oil
3 large cloves garlic, washed, peeled, and crushed but still intact

*Procedure*

- Measure olive oil into a small, heavy saucepan.
- Add crushed cloves of garlic.
- Cook over medium heat until small bubbles rise vigorously from the garlic.
- Remove from heat. Garlic will continue to cook.
- Allow garlic and oil to cool for a few minutes.
- Pour garlic and oil into a freshly washed glass jar with a lid.
- Remove the garlic from the oil after 24 hours.
- Store oil in the refrigerator for up to a week.

Yield: ½ C.

## Pecan Pie Granola Bars

Pre-wrapped "bars" have become a staple of modern life. I am often asked to suggest a FODMAP friendly bar, but most commercial fiber, protein, energy, nutrition, or snack bars are loaded with FODMAPs. Here is an easy recipe for a homemade bar that will fit the bill, made with wholesome and delicious ingredients, suitable for breakfast on the run or the lunch box. Something super sticky is needed to hold granola bars together— there's a reason why most commercial bars are made with honey or high-fructose corn syrup. Luckily, Karo light corn syrup and Lyle's Golden Syrup are suitable for use on the FODMAP Elimination Phase.

2 C. rolled oats
½ C. almond flour
½ C. oat flour
½ C. pumpkin seeds/pepitas, raw
1 C. chopped pecans
⅓ C. light corn syrup or golden syrup
1 large egg, beaten
⅓ C. oil
⅓ C. butter
1 T. vanilla

*Procedure*

- Preheat oven to 325° F and grease a large cookie tray with butter.
- Combine all ingredients in a medium size mixing bowl until thoroughly mixed, using hands or a wooden spoon.
- Transfer the dough to the cookie tray and pat it down into an even layer about ½ inch thick. Leave a little room around the edges, to make removal from the pan a little easier.
- Bake for 30 to 35 minutes, until brown around the edges. Dough might still be slightly soft in the middle.
- Allow bars to cool completely in the pan before cutting into 16 pieces.
- Place each bar in a sandwich-sized zip lock bag and store at room temperature.

*Recipe Tips*

- Make your own oat flour from rolled oats in seconds with a blender or food processor.
- Maple syrup can be used, but results in a softer, crumbly bar that burns easily.
- Use whatever nuts and seeds you have on hand (except pistachios for a total of 1¼ C.
- If you like the crispy edges best, use two cookie trays and divide the dough into 16 cookie-shaped patties. Reduce baking time as needed.

Servings: 16

**Peanut Butter Cookies**

Easy and delicious! This is everyone's favorite no-flour cookie.

1 large egg
1 C. natural peanut butter, smooth or chunky
1 C. granulated sugar

*Procedure*

- Preheat the oven to 350° F.
- Combine all ingredients in a mixing bowl.
- Form into ¾-inch balls or drop by slightly rounded teaspoons onto an ungreased cookie sheet.
- Dip the tines of a fork into the dough, then into some loose sugar in a small bowl.
- Press the back of the sugared fork into the dough to make a crisscross design on top of each cookie, flattening each one to approximately ¼ inch thick. Dip the back of the fork into the loose sugar in between pressing on each cookie.
- Bake 10-12 minutes, until the cookies look dry on top. Let the cookies cool on the cookie sheets before removing and storing in an airtight container. Makes 32 small cookies.

Servings: 16

**Lemon Vinaigrette Salad Dressing**

Simple! This delightful salad dressing lets the goodness of your fresh produce shine through.

2 medium lemons, juiced
6 T. extra virgin olive oil
1 t. maple syrup
½ t. sea salt
½ t. fresh-ground black pepper

*Procedure*

- Combine all ingredients in a glass jar. Shake well.
- Chill until serving.

Servings: 8

## Quinoa Salad

This mint and lemon-kissed recipe was contributed by Laura Molgaard. Quinoa is a very versatile, starchy seed that can be prepared in much the same way as rice and served hot or cold. It is high in protein and fiber.

2 C. quinoa, dry
4 C. water
1 large red bell pepper seeded & cut into ¼ inch cubes
zest of one lemon
juice of one lemon
¼ C. olive oil
1 T. sugar (or less, to taste)
½ t. salt
¼ t. freshly-ground black pepper
3 T. snipped chives or scallions/green onions (green part only)
½ C. chopped fresh mint or parsley

*Procedure*

- Measure quinoa into a medium saucepan, rinse thoroughly, and add 4 C. water.
- Bring to a boil over medium high heat, turn down to simmer, and cook until water is absorbed, approximately 15 minutes.
- Remove from heat and set aside to cool.
- Combine lemon zest, lemon juice, olive oil, sugar, salt, and pepper in a small bowl.
- Toss together cooled quinoa, chopped red pepper, dressing, chives, and mint.
- Adjust seasonings and serve warm or chilled.

*Recipe Tips*

- Unless you are certain the quinoa has been pre-rinsed, do it yourself. Rinsing removes the naturally occurring soap-like saponins from the quinoa and will improve its taste.
- Save money by purchasing dry quinoa in bulk; store at home in an airtight container.
-

Servings: 10

## Pork Fried Rice

This recipe is a great way to use up leftovers! When I cook rice for dinner, I often make extra in anticipation of making this family favorite the next night.

2 T. oil, divided
2 large eggs, lightly beaten
4 T. low-sodium soy sauce
2 ½ T. peanut butter
1 T. brown sugar, packed
1 T. rice (or other) vinegar
1 T. garlic oil
2 t. sesame oil, dark or spicy
¼ t. black pepper, freshly ground
hot sauce to taste
1 T. fresh ginger, peeled and minced
1 C. carrots, peeled and shredded
½ C. celery, chopped
4 C. rice, cooked, chilled
½ lb. pork, cooked and cubed
1 C. bean sprouts, fresh
1 C. pineapple chunks, drained
½ C. cashews
1 small bunch scallions, green part only, thinly sliced

*Procedure*

- Heat ½ T. oil over medium high heat in a large non-stick skillet.
- Add the eggs and cook, stirring constantly with a wooden or silicone spoon, until firm but not browned. Set aside.
- In a separate bowl, combine soy sauce, peanut butter, brown sugar, rice vinegar, garlic oil, sesame oil, black pepper, and hot sauce. Set aside.
- Heat remaining oil in the skillet until it spatters when a drop of water is dropped in the pan.
- Add ginger, carrots, and celery to the pan and sauté until tender.
- Transfer the chilled rice to the skillet and cook, stirring occasionally, for 5-10 minutes until it is heated through and slightly crispy in parts.

- Add remaining ingredients and prepared sauce, and continue to cook, stirring occasionally until everything is heated through.
- Serve immediately.

*Recipe Tips*

- Any kind of cooked meat, poultry, tofu or seafood can be substituted for the pork in this recipe.
- Short on time for veggie prep? Buy exactly the amounts you need from the grocery store salad bar.

Servings: 5

**Lactose-Free Yogurt**

I didn't use lactose-free yogurt in the sample menus because it is hard to find, but you can make your own lactose-free yogurt! You will have to purchase an inexpensive yogurt maker (appliance) for this recipe. A quick-read, digital or candy thermometer is also helpful to have on hand.

1 quart lactose-free, low-fat
1 packet freeze-dried yogurt starter

*Procedure*

- Pour the milk into a microwave-safe glass measuring cup or bowl.
- Heat the milk in a microwave oven on high for about seven minutes. Milk should be approximately 180°F. If you don't have a thermometer, look for steaming milk with bubbles around the edges. Do not boil the milk.
- Cool the milk until it is 115°F. This may take an hour or more, depending on the ambient temperature in the kitchen. If it accidentally gets too cool, re-warm it to 115°F.
- Combine the freeze-dried yogurt starter with approximately ½ C. of the warm milk in a separate cup. Stir with a spoon to combine well. Pour this mixture back into the large bowl of warm milk.
- Transfer the milk mixture to the incubation container of the electric yogurt maker and allow the yogurt to ferment according to the timing guidelines provided by the manufacturer of the yogurt starter, approximately 4-8 hours.
- The finished yogurt may show some separation of curds and whey.
- Refrigerate.
- Whey can be stirred back into the yogurt before serving, or strained off with a yogurt sieve or cheesecloth for a Greek-style yogurt.
- Sweeten the yogurt with a little maple syrup or sugar-sweetened jam before serving, if desired.

*Recipe Tips*

- If freeze-dried yogurt starter isn't available, you can use 2 T. of plain store-bought yogurt with live yogurt cultures instead. Make sure the yogurt doesn't have any pectin or other thickeners in it.
- In my 68° F kitchen, it takes 1 hour and 30 minutes for the hot milk to cool to 115° F.

Yield: 1 quart

**Chicken Seitan**

Seitan is a high-protein meat substitute made from wheat gluten. Use chicken seitan as a vegan protein in any of your favorite recipes. Seitan is included in this small recipe collection in case you wish to see what happens if you eat almost pure gluten outside of the wheat/rye/barley grain. Do not eat seitan if you have celiac disease or you are certain you have non-celiac gluten sensitivity.

10 oz. box vital wheat gluten
1 T. Bell's poultry seasoning
¼ t. garlic oil or olive oil
⅓ C. low-sodium soy sauce or water
2 C. water
8 C. water
¼ C. scallions, green part only, thinly sliced
⅛ t. black pepper freshly ground

*Procedure*

- Mix vital wheat gluten, Bell's poultry seasoning and garlic oil in a large glass bowl. Stir until very uniform mixture is formed.
- Combine ⅓ C. low-sodium soy sauce and 2 C. of water in a separate bowl.
- Pour liquid mixture into the gluten and stir until gluten develops into a rubbery ball.
- Remove the dough from the bowl and place it on a clean countertop.
- Knead the dough for a few minutes and shape into a log.
- Set the dough aside for 15 minutes while making the stock.
- Bring leftover soy sauce broth, 8 C. of water, scallions, and black pepper to a boil in a large stockpot.
- Cut the log of gluten into desired shapes and drop the gluten pieces into the boiling stock.
- Reduce heat to low, cover, and simmer for 45 minutes.
- Remove seitan from stock to a plate to cool. Refrigerate or freeze until serving.

Servings: 12

# BIBLIOGRAPHY AND RECOMMENDED READING

Akbar A, Yiangou Y, Facer P, Walters JRF, Anand P, Ghosh S. Increased capsaicin receptor TRPV1-expressing sensory fibres in irritable bowel syndrome and their correlation with abdominal pain. Gut 2008;57:923-929.

Arrigoni E, Brouns F, Amadò. Human gut microbiota does not ferment erythritol. Brit J Nutr 2005;94:643-646.

Austin GL, Dalton CB, Yuming H, Morris CB, Hankins J, Weinland SR, Westman EC, Yancy WS, Drossman DA. A very low-carbohydrate diet improves symptoms and quality of life in diarrhea-predominant irritable bowel syndrome. Clin Gastr Hepatol 2009;7(6):706-708.

Barret JS, Gibson PR. Development and validation of a comprensive semi-quantitative food frequency questionnaire that includes FODMAP intake and glycemic index. J Am Diet Assoc 2010;110:1469-1476.

Barrett JS, Gearry RB, Muir JG, Irving PM, Rose R, Rosella O, Haines ML, Shepherd SJ, Gibson PR. Dietary poorly absorbed, short-chain carbohydrates increase delivery of water and fermentable substrates to the proximal colon. Aliment Pharm Ther 2010 31:874-822.

Barrett JS, Gibson PR. Clinical ramifications of malabsorption of fructose and other short-chain carbohydrates. Pract Gastroenterol. 2007;51-65.

Barrett JS, Irving PM, Shepherd SJ, Muir JG, Gibson PR. Comparison of the prevalence of fructose and lactose malabsoption across chronic intestinal disorders. Aliment Pharm Ther 2009;30:165-174.

Beyer PL, Caviar EM, McCallum RW. Fructose intake at current levels in the United States may cause gastrointestinal distress in normal adults. J Am Diet Assoc. 2005 Oct;105:1559-1566.

Biesiekierski JR, Newnham ED, Irving PM, Garrett JS, Haines M, Doecke JD, Shepherd SJ, Muir JG, Gibson PR. Gluten causes gastrointestinal symptoms in subjects without celiac disease: A double-blind randomized placebo-controlled trial. Am J Gastroenterol 2011;106:508-514.

Biesiekierski JR, Rosella O, Rose R, Liels K, Barrett JS, Shepherd SJ, Gibson PR, Muir JG. Quantification of fructans, galacto-oligosaccharides and other short-chain carbohydrates in processed grains and cereals. J Hum Nutr Diet 2011 24(2):154-176.

Bijkerk CJ, de Wit NJ, Muris JWM, Whorwell PJ, Knottnerus JA, Hoes AW. Soluble or insoluble fibre in irritable bowel syndrome in primary care? Randomised placebo controlled trial. *BMJ 2009;339:b3154*

Bonnema AL, Kolber LW, Thomas W, Slavin JL. Gastrointestinal tolerance of chicory inulin Products. J Am Diet Assoc 2010;110:865-868.

Born P. Carbohydrate malabsorption in patients with non-specific abdominal complaints. World J Gastroenterol 2007; 13(43):5687-5691.

Brown LS, Current N. Not so sweet: Fructose malabsorption. Today's Dietitian 2011;13(9):70.

Camilleri M. Probiotics and Irritable Bowel Syndrome: Rationale, putative mechanisms, and evidence of clinical efficacy. J Clin Gastroenterol. 2006;40:264-269.

Camilleri M. Probiotics and irritable bowel syndrome: Rationale, mechanisms, and efficacy. J Clin Gastroeneterol 2008;42:S123-S125.

Chatterjee S, Park S, Low K, Kong Y, Pimentel M. The degree of breath methane production in IBS correlates with the severity of constipation. Am J Gastroenterol. 2007 Apr;102(4):837-841.

Cheng C, Bian Z, Zhu, L, Wu J, Sung J. Efficacy of a Chinese herbal proprietary medicine (Hemp Seed Pill) for functional constipation. Amer J Gastr 2011;106:120-129.

Chinda D, Nakaji S, Fukuda S, Sakamoto J, Shimoyama T, Nakamura T, Fujisawa T, Terada A, Sugawara K. Fermentation of different dietary fibers is associated with fecal clostridia levels in men. J Nutr 2004;134:1881-1886.

Choi CH, Jo SY, Park HJ, Chang SK, Byeon J, Myung S. A randomized, double-blind, placebo-controlled multicenter trial of saccharomyces boulardii in irritable bowel syndrome: Effect on quality of life. J Clin Gastroenterol 2011 Sep;45(8):679-683.

Choi YK, Johlin FC, Summers RW, Jackson M, Rao SC. Fructose intolerance: an under-recognized problem. Am J Gastr 2003;98(6):1348-1353.

Christie C, ed. The Florida Medical Nutrition Therapy Manual, (Florida Dietetic Association) 2005. P. 4.1-4.2.

Cremon C, Gargano L, Morselli-Labate AM, Santini D, Cogliandro RF, De Giorgio R, Stanghellini V, Corinaldesi R, Barbara G. Mucosal immune activation in irritable bowel syndrome: Gender-dependence and association with digestive symptoms. Amer J Gastr 2009;104:392-400.

Croagh C, Shepherd SJ, Merryman M, Muir JG, Gibson PR. Pilot study on the effect of reducing dietary FODMAP intake on bowel function in patients without a colon. Inflamm Bowel Dis 2007;12:1522-1528.

Cummings JH, MacFarlane GT, Englyst HN. Prebiotic digestion and fermentation. Am J Clin Nutr 2001;73:415S-20S.

Dean BB, Aguilar D, Barghout V, Kahler KH, Frech F, Groves D, Ofman J. Impairment in work productivity and health-related quality of life in patients with IBS. Am J Manag C 2005;11(1):S17-26.

DeVries J, Post B, Medallian Laboratories. Polydextrose technical bulletin. Retrieved October 23, 2011 from http://www.medlabs.com/Downloads/polydextrose.pdf.

Dunlop SP, Hebden J, Campbell E, Naesdal J, Olbe L, Perkins AC, Spiller RC. Abnormal intestinal permeability in subgroups of diarrhea-predominant irritable bowel syndromes. Am J Gastroenterol 2006;101:1288-1294.

Eadala P, Waud JP, Matthews SB, Green JT, Campbell AK. Quantifying the 'hidden' lactose in drugs used for the treatment of gastrointestinal conditions. Aliment Pharmacol Ther 2009;15(6):677-687.

Eastern Health Cinical School—Monash University. *The Low FODMAP Diet; Reducing Poorly Absorbed Sugars to Control Gastrointestinal Symptoms* (booklet). Monash University, Victoria, Australia, 2011.

Electronic Code of Federal Regulations, Title 21 Food and Drugs, Section 101.9. Retrieved November 18, 2011 from http://ecfr.gpoaccess.gov/cgi/t/text/text-idx?c=ecfr;rgn=div5;view=text;node=21%3A2.0.1.1.2;idno=21;sid=64fa2cdef4ee54e80414c2f297540271;cc=ecfr.

Emmanuel AV, Tack J, Quigley EM, Talley NJ. Pharmacological management of constipation. Neurogastroenterol Motil 2009;21(Suppl.2):41-54.

Eswaran S, Tack J, Chey WD. Food: The forgotten factor in the irritable bowel syndrome. Clin N Amer 2011(40):141-162.

Food and Agrigulture Organization of the United Nations. *Carbohydrates in Human Nutrition, Report of a Joint FAO/WHO Consultation*, Rome. April 1997. Retrieved October 23, 2011 from http://www.fao.org/docrep/W8079E/w8079e00.HTM

Ford AC, Chey WD, Talley NJ, Malhotra A, Spiegel MR, Moayyedi P. Yield of diagnostic tests for celiac disease in individuals with symptoms suggestive of irritable bowel syndrome. Arch Intern Med 2009; 169(7):651-658.

Ford AC, Talley NJ, Spiegel BMR, Foxx-Orenstein AE, Schiller L, Quigley EMM, Moayyedi P. Effect of fibre, antispasmodics, and peppermint oil in the treatment of irritable bowel syndrome: systemic review and meta-analysis. Brit Med J 2008;13:3370:237-246.

Francavilla R, Miniello V, Magistà AM, De Canio A, Bucci N, Gagliardi F, Lionetti E, Castellaneta S, Polimeno L, Peccarisi L, Intrio F, Cavallo L. A Randomized Controlled Trial of Lactobacillus GG in Children With Functional Abdominal Pain. Pediatrics 2010;126;e1445-e1452.

Gearry RB, Irving PM, Nathan DM, Barrett JS, Shepherd SJ, Gibson PR. The effect of reduction of poorly absorbed, highly fermentable short chain carbohydrates (FODMAPs) on the symptoms of patients with inflammatory bowel disease (IBD). J Gastroen Hepatol. 2007;22(supp 3):A292.

Gibson PR, Shepher SJ. Evidence-based Dietary Management of Functional Gastrointestinal Symptoms: The FODMAP Approach. J Gastroenterol Hepatol. 2010;25(2):252-258.

Gibson PR, Shepherd SJ. Evidence-based dietary management of functional gastrointestinal symptoms: the FODMAP approach. J Gastr Hepatol 2010;25(2):252-258.

Goldstein R, Braverman D, Stankiewicz H. Carbohydrate malabsorption and the effect of dietary restriction on symptoms of irritable bowel syndrome and functional bowel complaints. Isr Med Assoc J 2000;2:583-587.

Grabitske HA, Slavin JL. Gastrointestinal effects of low-digestible carbohydrates. Crit Rev Food Sci Nutr 2009,49(4):327-360.

Granito M, Frias J, Doblado R, Guerra M, Champ M, Vidal-Valverde C. Nutritional improvement of beans (Phaseolus vulgaris) by natural fermentation. Eur Food Res Technol 2002;214:226-231.

Gwee K. Fiber, FODMAPs, flora, flatulence and the functional bowel disorders. J Gastroenterol Hepatol. 2010 25:1335-1336.

Hadley SK, Gaarder SM. Treatment of irritable bowel syndrome. Am Fam Physician. 2005 Dec;72(12):2501-2506.

Halpert A, Dalton CB, Palsson O, Morris C, Hu Y, Bangkiwala S, Hankins J, Norton N. What patients know about irritable bowel syndrome (IBS) and what they would like to know. National survey on patient educational needs in IBS and development and validation of the Patient Educational Needs Questionnaire (PEQ). Amer J Gastr 2007;102:1972-1982.

Hanover ML, White JS. Manufacturing, composition and applications of fructose. Am J Clin Nutr.1993;58(suppl):724S-32S.

Health Canada. Sugar alcohols (polyols) and polydextrose used as sweeteners in food. 2005. Retrieved October 23, 2011 from http://www.hc-sc.gc.ca/fn-an/securit/addit/sweeten-edulcor/polyols_polydextose_factsheet-polyols_polydextose_fiche-eng.php.

Heizer WD, Southern S, McGovern S. The role of diet in symptoms of irritable bowel syndrome in adults: a narrative review. J Amer Diet Assoc 2009;1091204-1214.

Hoekstra JH, van den Aker JHL. Facilitating effect of amino acids on fructose and sorbitol absorption in children. J Pediatr Gastr Nutr 1996;23(2):118-124.

Imperial Malts, Ltd. Retrieved December 28, 2011 from http://www.imperialmalt.com/malt-extract.html.

Inadomi JM, Fennerty MB, Bjorkman D. The economic impact of irritable bowel syndrome. Aliment Pharmacol Ther 2003;28(7):671-682.

International Organics, Energave. Raw, organic agave nectar, 2008. Retrieved November 13, 2011 at http://www.international-organics.com/info-files/Intl_Organics_Organic_Agave_Info.pdf.

Jiménez MB. Treatment of irritable bowel syndrome with probiotics. An etiopathogenic approach at last? Rev Esp Enferm Dig 2009;101(8):553-564.

Karppinen S, Myllymäki O, Forssell P, Poutanen K. Fructan Content of Rye and Rye Products. Cereal Chem 2003;80(2):168–171.

Karppinen S. Dietary fibre components of rye bran and their fermentation in vitro. Espoo 2003. VTT Publications 500. Retrieved October 26, 2011 at http://ethesis.helsinki.fi/julkaisut/bio/bioja/vk/karppinen/dietar yf.pdf.

Kolfenbach L. The pathophysiology, diagnosis and treatment of IBS. J Amer Acad Phys Assist. 2007 Jan;(20)1:16-20.

Lavender, R. Following the ripening of bananas. Chem Sci. 2006 Feb;3 Retrieved October 23, 2011 from http://www.rsc.org/Publishing/ChemScience/Volume/2006/03/ ripening_of_bananas.asp.

Leavitt MD, Duane WC. Floating stools—flatus versus fat. New Engl J Med 1972;286(18)973-975.

Ledochowski M, Sperner-Unterweger B, Fuchs D. Lactose malabsorption is associated with early signs of mental depression in females. A preliminary report. J Dig Dis 1998; 43(11)2513-2517.

Ledochowski M, Überall F, Propst T, Fuchs D, Fructose malabsorption is associated with lower plasma folic acid concentrations in middle-aged subjects. Clin Chem 1999;45(11):2013-2014.

Ledochowski M, Widner B, Bair H, Probst T, Fuchs D. Fructose- and sorbitol-reduced diet improves mood and gastrointestinal disturbance in fructose malabsorbers. Scand J Gastr 2000;35:1048-1052.

Ledochowski M, Widner B, Murr C, Fuchs D, Decreased serum zinc in fructose malabsorbers. Clin Chem 2001;47(4):745- 747.

Lee CY, Shallenberger RS, Vittum MT. Free sugars in fruits and vegetables. New York's Food and Life Sciences Bulletin. 1970;1:1-12.

Levine BL, Weisman S. Enzyme replacement as an effective treatment for the common symptoms of complex carbohyrdrate intolerance. Nutr Clin Care 2004;7(2):75-81.

Lifeway Foods. 411 on Lactose Intolerance and Lifeway Kefir. Retrieved December 1, 2011 from http://lifeway.net/Portals/1/lactoseintolerance.pdf.

Macfarlane GT, Steed H, Macfarlane SJ. Bacterial metabolism and health-related effects of glacto-oligosaccharides and other prebiotics. Appl Microbiol 2008;104(2):305-344.

Maxion-Bergemann S, Thielecke E, Abel E, Bergemann R. Costs of irritable bowel syndrome in the UK and US. Pharmacoeconomics 2006;24(1):21-37.

McCleary BV, Murphy A. Measurement of total fructan in foods by enzymatic/spectrophotometric methods: Collaborative study. J AOAC Int 2000;83(2):356-364.

Morcos A, Dinan T, Quigley EMM. Irritable bowel syndrome: Role of food in pathogenesis and management. J Digest Dis 2009;10(4):237-246.

Moshfegh, AJ, Friday JE, Goldman JP, Chug A, Jaspreet K. Presence of inulin and oligofructose in the diets of Americans, J Nutr. 1999;129:1407S-1411S.

Muir JG, Shepherd SJ, Rosella O, Rose R, Barrett JS, Gibson PR. Fructan and free fructose content of common Australian vegetables and fruit. J Agric Food Chem 2007;55:6619-6627.

Nathan DM, Shepherd SJ, Berryman M, Muir JG, Iser JH, Gibson PR. Fructose malabsorption in Crohn's disease: a common contributor to symptoms that benefit from dietary modification. J Gastroen Hepatol. 2005;20(Suppl.):A27.

National Kefir Association. Retrieved January 8, 2012 from http://nationalkefirassociation.com.

National Starch and Chemical Company, About RS – Resistant Starch. Retrieved December 29, 2011 from http://www.resistantstarch.com/ResistantStarch/About+RS/.

National Yogurt Association. Retrieved January 8, 2012 from http://www.aboutyogurt.com.

Neal KR, Hebden J, Spiller R. Prevalence of gastrointestinal symptoms six months after bacterial gastroenteritis and risk factors for development of the irritable bowel syndrome: postal survey of patients. Brit Med J 1997;314(7083):779-782.

Niness KR. Inulin and oligofructose: What are they? J Nutr. 1999; 129:1402S-1406S.

Nucera G, Gabrielli M, Lupascu A, Lauritano EC, Santoliquido A, Cremonini F, Cammarota G, Tondi P, Pola P, Gasbarrini G, Gasbarrini A. Abnormal breath tests to lactose, fructose and sorbitol in irritable bowel syndrome may be explained by small intestinal bacterial overgrowth. Aliment Pharm Therap. 2005;21(11):1391-1395.

Oklahoma Cooperative Extension Service. Let's compare dairy goats and cows. Retrieved November 18, 2011 from http://ansi4900.okstate.edu/youth%20extension/files/dairy.goats.cows.pdf.

Ong DK, Shaylyn M, Barrett JS, Shepherd SJ, Irving PM, Biesiekierski J, Smith S, Gibson PR, Muir JG. Manipulation of dietary short chain carbohydrates alters the pattern of gas production and genesis of symptoms in irritable bowel syndrome. J Gastroen Hepatol 2010 25:1366-1373.

Parkes GC, Brostoff J, Whelan K, Sanderson JD. Gastrointesitnal microbiota in irritable bowel syndrome: Their role in its pathogenesis and treatment. Am J Gastroenterol 2008;103:1557-1567.

Pimentel M, Lembo A, Chey WD, Zakko S, Ringel Y, Yu J, Mareya SM, Shaw AL, Bortey E, Forbes WP for the TARGET Study Group, Rifaximin therapy for patients with irritable bowel wyndrome without constipation. N Engl J Med 2011:364:22-32.

Purdue University Center for New Plants and Plant Products. Retricved December 29, 2011 from http://www.hort.purdue.edu/newcrop/crops/corn.html

Prosky L, Hoebregs H. Methods to determine food inulin and oligofructose. J Nutr 1999;129:1418S-1423S.

Quigley, EMM. Probiotics in irritable bowel syndrome: An immunomodulatory strategy? J Am Coll Nutr 2007;26(6):684S-690S.

Rackis JJ. Flatulence caused by soya and its control through processing. J Am Oil Chem Soc 1981;58(3):503-510.

Rao SC, Attaluri A, Anderson L, Stumbo P. The ability of the normal human small intestine to absorb fructose: Evaluation by breath testing. Clin Gastr Hepatol 2007;5(8):958-963.

Rumessen, JJ, Gudmand-Høyer E. Fructans of chicory: Intestinal transport and fermentation of different chain lengths and relation to fructose and sorbitol malabsorption. Am J Clin Nutr 1998;68:357–364.

Scarlata, K. The Complete Idiot's Guide to Eating Well with IBS, Alpha Books, USA, 2010.

SCIOTEC Diagnostic Technologies, Scientific information on fructose malabsorption & FRUCTOSIN. Retrieved November 18, 2011 from http://www.google.com/url?sa=t&rct=j&q=&esrc=s&source=we b&cd=1&ved=0CB4QFjAA&url=http%3A%2F%2Fshop.alles-essen.at%2Fjoom_en%2Findex.php%3Foption%3Dcom_joomdo c%26task%3Ddoc_download%26gid%3D20%26Itemid%3D2%26 lang%3Dde&ei=e9sJT-TZAebn0QHbwPXJAg&usg=AFQjCNGvSToK9xZ6cPeN9gzgiR jgWum3uA.

Shaheen NJ, Hansen RA, Morgan DR, Gangarosa LM, Ringel Y, Thiny MR, Russo MW, Sandler RS. The burden of gastrointestinal and liver diseases, 2006. Am J Gastroenterol 2006;101:2128-2137.

Shepherd SJ, Parker FC, Muir JG, Gibson PR. Dietary triggers of abdominal symptoms in patients with irritable bowel syndrome: randomized placebo-controlled evidence. Clin Gastr Hepatol 2008;6:765-771.

Shepherd, SJ, Shepherd Works. Retrieved January 8, 2012 from www.shepherdworks.com.au.

Signet Diagnostic Corporation. Leap-Disease Management Website. Retrieved January 8, 2012 from http://www.nowleap.com/.

Simrén M, Axelsson J, Gillberg R, Abrahamsson H, Svedlund J, Björnsson ES. Quality of life in inflammatory bowel disease in remission: The impact of IBS-like symptoms and associated psychological factors. Am J Gastroenterol. 2002 Feb;97(2):389-396.

Spiller R, Postinfectious functional dyspepsia and postinfectious irritable bowel syndrome: different symptoms but similar risk factors. Gastroenterology 2010;138(5):1600-1663.

Stone-Dorshow T, Levitt MD. Gaseous response to ingestion of a poorly absorbed fructo-oligosaccharide sweetener. Am J Clin Nutr. 1987;46:61-65.

Suares NC, Ford AC. Systemic review: the effects of fibre in the management of chronic idiopathic constipation. Aliment Pharmacol Ther 2011;33(8):895-901.

The Sugar Association, Inc. Retrieved January 8, 2012 from http://www.sugar.org.

Thiwan S. Lactose intolerance and small bowel bacterial overgrowth in irritable bowel syndrome. The UNC Center for Functional GI and Motility Disorders. Retrieved October 23, 2011 from http://www.med.unc.edu/ibs/files/educational-gi-handouts/Abdominal%20Bloating.pdf/at_download/file.

Thiwan, Sayed, MD. Abdominal bloating: A mysterious symptom. Retrieved November 13, 2011 at http://www.med.unc.edu/ibs/files/educational-gi-handouts/Abdominal%20Bloating.pdf.

Tomlin DJ, Read NW. The effect of feeding xanthan gum on colonic function in man: Correlation with in vitro determinants of bacterial breakdown. Brit J Nutr 1993;69:897-902.

Tosh SM, Yada S. Dietary fibres in pulse seeds and fractions: Characterization, functional attributes, and applications. Food Research International 2010;43:450-460.

Tungland BC, Meyer D. Nondigestible olig- and polysaccharides (dietary fiber): their physiology and role in human health and food. Compr Rev Food Sci F. 2002;1:73-92.

Van de Meulen R, Scheirlinck I, Van Schoor A, Huys G, Vancanneyt M, Vandamme P, De Vuyst L. Population dynamics and metabolite target analysis of lactic acid bacteria during laboratory fermentations of wheat and spelt sourdoughs. Appl Environ Microb 2007;73(15):4741-4750.

Varea V, de Carpi JM, Puig C, Alda JA, Camacho E, Ormazabal A, Artuch R, Gómez L. Malabsorption of Carbohydrates and Depression in Children and Adolescents. J Pediatr Gastr Nutr 40:561-565.

Ventura EE, Davis JN, Goran MI. Sugar content of popular sweetened beverages based on objective laboraroy analysis: Focus on fructose content. Obesity 2011;4:868-874.

Verdu EF, Armstron DA, Murray JA. Between celiac disease and irritable bowel syndrome: The "no man's land" of gluten sensitivity. Am J Gastroenterol 2009;104:1587-1594.

Verdu EF. Can gluten contribute to irritable bowel syndrome? Am J Gastroenterol 2011;106:516-518.

Vos MB, Kimmons JE, Gillespie C, Welsh J, Blanck HM. Dietary fructose consumption among US children and adults: the Third National Health and Nutrition Examination Survey, Medscape J Med. 2008;10(7):160. Retrieved October 23, 2011 from http://www.medscape.com/viewarticle/576945.

Whelan K, Abrahmsohn O, David GJP, Staudacher H, Irving P, Lomer MCE, Ellis PR. Fructan content of commonly consumed wheat, rye and gluten-free breads. Int J Food Sci Nutr 2011 62(5):498-503.

Whey Protein Institute. Whey Protein FAQ. Retrieved October 23, 2011 from http://www.wheyoflife.org/faq.cfm.

Wilt TJ, Shaukat A, Shamliyan T, Taylor BC, MacDonald R, Tacklind J, Rutks I, Schwarzenberg SJ, Kane RL, and Levitt M. Lactose Intolerance and Health. No. 192 (Prepared by the Minnesota Evidence-based Practice Center under Contract No. HHSA 290-2007-10064-I.) AHRQ Publication No. 10-E004. Rockville, MD. Agency for Healthcare Research and Quality. February 2010.

Zörb C, Betsche T, Langenkämper G, Zapp J, Seifert M. Free Sugars in spelt wholemeal and flour. J Appl Bot Food Qual 2007;81:172-174

## ACKNOWLEDGEMENTS

I am blessed with a wonderful family, remarkable patients and colleagues, and an interactive world-wide community of readers.

My husband Paul has been supportive of this project from day one; knowing that he believed in me 100% was all the encouragement I needed to begin. I would like to thank my daughter Laura Catsos for testing and editing some of the recipes in this book, and my daughter Christine Catsos for editorial assistance with the manuscript. My brother, Paul Danehy, and my brother-in-law Gregg Sauter, have been especially generous with their time, coaching me on some of the business aspects of my publishing endeavors.

When I finished the first edition of this book, I felt a tremendous sense of relief and accomplishment! But I soon realized that it was only the beginning of my journey with FODMAPs. My clients, book readers, blog readers, Twitter and Facebook followers are an eager audience. Each note, comment, and tweet challenges me to read more, learn more, and share more. I truly consider my patients, readers, and followers collaborators in this work. Without you, this second edition would not have been possible.

I would like to thank many colleagues both near and far who challenge me with their questions, share resources, and help spread the word about FODMAPs, especially the members of the Academy of Nutrition and Dietetics' Nutrition Entrepreneurs Dietetic Practice Group. I also value my colleagues on the Certified LEAP Therapist Listserv. I particularly enjoy collaboration with Kate Scarlata, RD, LDN, another FODMAP champion and author of *The Complete Idiot's Guide to Eating Well with IBS* (Alpha, 2010). Niki Strealy, RD, LD (author of The Diarrhea Dietitian: Expert Advice, Practical Solutions and Strategic Nutrition) and  Carol Ireton-Jones, PhD, RD, LD, CNSC (consultant in private practice and Managing Partner, Professional Nutrition Therapists, Dallas, Texas) were kind enough to serve as advance readers and reviewers of my manuscript.

I greatly appreciate and admire Susan Quimby, RD, LD, and the rest of my colleagues at Nutrition Works, LLC in Portland, Maine. Susan has been so very generous with her support and encouragement of this aspect of my practice. Kitty Broihier, MS, RD, co-author of several cookbooks including *The Everyday Low-Carb Slow Cooker Cookbook* (De Capo Press, 2004), provided valuable advice and encouragement as I weighed the merits of self-publishing vs. traditional publishing models. Jillian Smith, nutrition student at the University of New Hampshire, assisted with research, recipe development and testing, and writing some guest blog posts to help vegans and vegetarians navigate the diet. Jennifer Caven provided copyediting services, though as a self-published author, I take full responsibility for any errors that remain in the text. My sincere thanks to all of you, and to anyone else I may have inadvertently omitted.

Readers, I look forward to continuing our FODMAP conversation at www.ibsfree.net and www.facebook.com/IBSFree.

## ABOUT THE AUTHOR

Patsy Danehy Catsos, M.S., R.D., L.D. is a nutritionist on a mission to reduce pain and improve quality of life for clients with gastrointestinal problems or food sensitivities. The days of over-generalized advice for people with stomach problem are over. "Eat more fiber" and "avoid red meat, alcohol, and caffeine" just don't cut it anymore. Patsy doesn't believe in one-size-fits-all diets; she helps you discover the diet that works for you!

Her trailblazing book, *IBS—Free at Last!* (Pond Cove Press, 2009), introduced U.S. health care providers and consumers to an exciting and effective dietary program for finding and eliminating food triggers for irritable bowel syndrome. Patsy is the editor of the blog IBSfree.net, and an expert contributor to Sharecare.com, an interactive social Q/A platform created by Jeff Arnold and Dr. Mehmet Oz in partnership with Harpo Studios, HSW International, Sony Pictures Television, and Discovery Communications. She has been consulted for expert comment in numerous publications, including *WebMD*, *Today's Dietitian*, and *Consumer Reports Shop Smart Magazine*.

Ms. Catsos earned a B.S. in Nutritional Science from Cornell University and an M.S. in Nutrition at Boston University. She completed her internship at Boston's Beth Israel Hospital. Ms. Catsos maintains a private practice in Portland, Maine. She is a professional member of the Crohn's and Colitis Foundation of American and the Academy of Nutrition and Dietetics (formerly known as the American Dietetic Association), as well as past-president of the Maine Dietetic Association.

Patsy looks forward to corresponding with readers through her blog, www.ibsfree.net. Use the "comments" link at the bottom of each blog post to ask questions, let her know how this book has helped you, or share information that might help others. She also welcomes your reviews on Amazon.com and other retail websites.

Follow @CatsosIBSFreeRD on Twitter or "like" facebook.com/IBSFree to be notified about new blog posts, FODMAP-friendly foods, and other items of interest.

# INDEX

food sources of, 78
malabsorption, 78
malabsorption of, 81, 83, 93
Carrots, 44
Casein, 122
Cauliflower, 66, 75, 89
Celery, 44
Celery seeds, 116
Celiac disease, 14, 16, 81, 85,
  130
Challenge
  fructans, 64
  fructose, part A, 62
  fructose, part B, 63
  galactans/GOS, 67
  lactose, 61
  polyols, 66
Challenge food lists, rank order
  of, 126
Challenge Phase, 57
  directions for, 57
  moderate symptoms, 126
  no symptoms, 125
  severe symptoms, 125, 126
  worksheet, 59
Cheese, 48
  lactose content of, 85
Cheeses, allowed, 48
Cherries, 66, 75
Cherry tomatoes, 44
Chewing gum, 66, 75, 89
Chia seeds, 95
Chick peas, 76
Chicken, 48
Chicken Seitan, recipe, 146
Chickpeas, 49, 67, 90
Chicory, 51
Chicory root extract, 40, 51, 53,
  64, 74, 88
Children, 71
Chili peppers, 44, 116
Chili powder, 116
Chips, allowed, 40
Chives, 44, 116
Chocolate, 52
Cilantro, 116
Cinnamon, 116
Citric acid, 91

Clementines, 42
Cocoa, 52
Coconut, 46, 50
Coffee, 50, 67, 76, 115
Conflicting information about
  FODMAPs, 104
Constipation, 82, 121
  during Elimination Phase,
    121
Contraindications, possible, 15,
  71
Coriander, 116
Corn, 40, 80, 104, 122
  sweet, 40, 66, 75, 89, 112
Corn starch, 41, 52
Corn sugar, 87
Corn syrup, 50, 87, 117
Cottage cheese, 48, 61, 73
Cough drops, 66, 75
Couscous, 64, 74
Cranberries, 42, 62, 74, 104
Cream, 46
Cream cheese, 46
Crohn's disease, 2, 9, 12, 13, 14,
  81, 85, 130
Crystalline fructose, 41, 43, 45,
  46, 50, 53, 62, 73
Cucumber, 44
Cultured corn syrup, 52
Cumin, 116
Dairy, 112
Dates, 66, 74, 75
Depression, 98
Dextrose, 52, 131
Dietary fiber
  classification of, 80
  definition of, 80, 93
  food sources of, 108
  getting enough of, 108
Dietary fructose intolerance, 93,
  133
Dietitian
  follow up with, 121
  how to find, 91
Digestive enzymes, 80, 81, 88,
  132
  deficiency of, 81
  lactase, 85

Made in the USA
San Bernardino, CA
24 January 2015